P9-DML-234

"Marti Matthews writes straight from my soul. I endorse her book 100%.

—**Dr. Elizabeth Kübler-Ross,** author of
On Death & Dying

"For those who are ready to heal their lives. This book helps us find our true path through God's redirections, and thus out of the pain comes a gift."

—**Dr. Bernie Siegel,** author of
Love, Medicine & Miracles

"Everyone in pain needs hope and inspiration. Marti Matthews provides both. I strongly recommend this book for all those who suffer."

—**Dr. C. Norman Shealy,** co-author of
Aids: Passageway to Transformation

"I like Marti's book for two reasons. One: as a man, I need help addressing the pain in my life. Two: because her book will help the ministry of care-givers anywhere."

—**Tom Mullen,** Dean Emeritus of
Earlham School of Religion

"A sensitive mix of poetry, prose, and confession. Marti Matthews seeks blessing in the paradox of grace. She knows that gift is always hidden in tragedy, and her words give hope to those who despair in the midst of life. A book for those who want to give up."

—**Dr. Stephen A. Schmidt,** author of
Living with Chronic Illness

"A challenge and an inspiration to anyone who has felt pain—and that's most of us. Whether the pain is physical or spiritual, this wise book will help us to understand and to grow."

—**Madeleine L'Engle,** author of
A Wrinkle in Time

PAIN

The Challenge & the Gift

MARTI LYNN MATTHEWS

STILLPOINT

STILLPOINT PUBLISHING

Building a society that honors the Earth,

Humanity, and the Sacred in all Life.

For a free catalog or ordering information, write
Stillpoint Publishing, Box 640, Walpole NH 03608 USA
or call
1-800-847-4014 TOLL FREE (Continental US, except NH)
1-603-756-9281 (Foreign and NH)

Copyright © 1991 Marti Lynn Matthews

All rights reserved. No part of this book may be reproduced without written permission from the publisher, except by a reviewer who may quote brief passages or
reproduce illustrations in a review; nor may any part of this book be reproduced,
stored in a retrieval system, or transmitted in any form or by any means electronic,
mechanical, photocopying, recording, or other, without written permission from the
publisher.

This book is manufactured in the United States of America.
Cover and text design by Karen Savary.

Published by Stillpoint Publishing, a division of Stillpoint International, Box 640,
Meetinghouse Road, Walpole, NH 03608.

Library of Congress Catalog Card Number: 91-065958

Matthews, Marti Lynn
Pain: The Challenge & the Gift

ISBN 0-913299-80-4

1 2 3 4 5 6 7 8 9 0

To my beloved Tom:
The joy of knowing you was worth the pain of parting.

O speak, you unheard voice of nature,
I'm ready to hear.
O tell me, where can Love be found in Pain?

Breathe through the heat of our desire
thy coolness and thy balm.
Let sense be dumb, let flesh retire;
speak through the earthquake, wind and fire,
O still small voice of calm!

—JOHN GREENLEAF WHITTIER

O tell me, where can Love be found in Pain?

Contents

VI: MOVING ON

Acknowledgments

There are people who take the heart out of you, and there are people who put it back.

—Elizabeth David

MANY PEOPLE MUST BE THANKED FOR THE BIRTH OF THIS book. I'm thankful for the sensitivity of my mother and the joie de vivre of my father, which live in me as their gifts. Although these were hard to bring into marriage inside me, they are the best parts of "me."

I'd like to thank all the dear friends and all the teachers and all the writers of books who've helped me grow through pain over the years. I thank my professors at Mundelein College in Chicago, who taught me to examine and think in depth. I thank an organization in the Chicago area called Common Ground, which helped me explore in an unrestricted way the thought of the world and introduced me to wholistic ways of thinking. I thank a particular professor, Kathy Tillman, who saw in me something much bigger than what I saw in myself.

I thank my beloved Quaker Meeting for being with me in sacred silence, where the Still Small Voice speaks to us regularly. I send a large hug to Limina, a Chicago educational and spiritual sisterhood that blessed and lifted up my womanhood to its proper nobility. I thank and bless my children, Tom and Anne Marie Dix, who encourage me and share ideas with me. I even thank anyone who's ever caused me pain—how rich my life is because of all that pain has given me! But I won't mention those people by name. . . .

Many friends have read and commented on parts of the manuscript. I mention especially those who I know gave much time and thought to this: Tom Martish, Felicia Kaplan, Hugh Barbour, Randy Bennet, Dave Garman, Tom Forsythe, and Lillith Quinlan, as well as all the friends whose stories or thoughts are quoted herein.

The reference librarians at Niles Public Library and the specialists at Skokie Public Library deserve special mention for their dedicated efforts to find sources that I collected in my haphazard manner, without remembering where I'd found them.

I'm grateful for the delightful experience of studying writing with Madeleine L'Engle at Mundelein College, and I appreciate her encouragement and advice.

I'm grateful to the Earlham School of Religion for granting me, in the spring of 1989, the John Patrick Henry Memorial Christian Writers' Scholarship, which enabled me to develop this manuscript, and to the person to whom I'm most indebted: Tom Mullen, Dean of the Earlham School of Religion, who gave me guidance and such warm and clear encouragement.

I feel thrilled and grateful to be working with the wonderful people at Stillpoint International, a publishing company that works not just for its own survival but with love and dedication to the world.

Introduction

LIFE IS SAFE AND SOLID. IT HAS TAKEN A LIFETIME, BUT I've finally become convinced of this.

The search of my life has been to find a certainty that even in the worst and most mysterious corners of life we are upheld, that the ground on which we walk is secure.

Pain is the shakiest part of any positive philosophy we try to believe in. All that is good seems betrayed by pain. But in the end, I've found pain to be solid. Pain is not a bad trick by a fickle force. Rather, pain is also love.

Until we become familiar with it, pain can seem a monster. Becoming familiar doesn't mean spending time with it. It means treating pain as we would a grouchy family member, a bitter relative who has come to live with us but is unwelcome. Must life be spoiled by this bitter element of our experience? How can we deal with it? What does it really want, and *why* is this sourness here? Can we be happy living in this shadow? Is there a way to get rid of it?

The problem-solving person watches the way this spoilsport functions, what its characteristics and its needs are. When pain speaks in its awful voice, what is it trying to say? And who will help me deal with this—am I alone in my problem?

My answer is no, and we have never been alone. The loving power that accompanies us from beginning to end I call Grace.

Grace is the womb in which we enter this world, and then it is the air we breathe, the earth that upholds us, the sunshine that follows us whether we're aware of it or not. We are surrounded and upheld by love and care, even in the storm. We cannot step out of the presence of Grace; we can only close our eyes to Its presence and ignore Its help.

Creation may first have been an idea and a word, but we are brought into this world through pain and effort and love. It is the Divine Mother who brings us into existence and who will stay with us and bring us to completion. Grace is with us in every moment, the fecund and powerful Mother of the World.

My own concept of the source of life is slightly different from the common idea of "God." While I believe clearly that we are not alone in life, that there is power and purpose surrounding our existence, that there is source and goal, I avoid the word "God" for several reasons. For me, it carries a very strong image: that of Michelangelo's old man in the sky reaching out to create—very male, very separate from a creation that he's finished. To me, rather, creation is always ongoing. Divine energy constantly bursts forth into creation, it upholds all, it is the very energy of life in all its forms. The Divine Energy is both female and male, personal and more than personal. It is the substance of every part and still greater than all Its parts.

To show the inseparable relationship between the Source of Life and the forms of life, I use many names: the Mother as well as the Father, Grace, All-That-Is, the Life Force or Life Energy, Love, Divine Love, Mercy, All-the-Power-in-the-Universe, and above all, the Beloved Source of Life.

* * *

The Beloved Source of Life is not unchanging but is always expanding through creation. God dreams a dream and we are born. But it is one thing to conceive an idea; it is something else to bring it to completion step by step. We are all still being created. We are groping toward wholeness, longing to finish the dream that's inside us. Grace knows how much it cost to begin us and will help us reach our wholeness, to be whatever we are trying so hard to become. We are loved and treasured, we are longed for and needed. All The-Power-in-the-Universe wants us to succeed. Grace upholds us, but we must do the work. We create ourselves and our world through our choices and effort.

To be clear with you: pain, for me, is also a face of God. It is the divine presence in our lives in a form we have not understood as love. I call it the Other, or the Ruthless Other. I hope in this book to help you see that pain is not separate from God; it is not a power in opposition to goodness. Pain is a sacrament, love in a form beyond the boundaries of our immediate understanding and expectations.

There are other, simpler ways to approach an understanding of pain. We could call it a "rule of the game," boundaries, a guide, a feedback system, a limit, a mirror. Pain is the teacher, our spirit guide, a gift-giver. Pain is the face of Divine Love that Hindus call "Kali," the goddess who destroys in order to create. The strong creative desire of Kali sweeps away the old ruthlessly to make way for the wonderful new.

Pain is never punishment. It is always opportunity. When we turn toward the opportunity, pain loses its sting and power. We must *accept* something, not put our effort into throwing it out. Often when we find and accept the gift in our pain, that pain can disappear. There is only one door, and that is to accept the gift our pain is trying to give us.

Even death is not a failure. It is the natural close of one

adventure. The healing of our pain and the receipt of its gift may be the completion of a learning, one that permits our soul to move on. Pain may be the guide who takes us out of the limits of time and into eternity, convincing us finally to go through the door.

By what authority do I speak?

Pain has been my guide most of my life, for better or for worse, necessary or unnecessary. I have known pain: physical, emotional, individual, group. I've come to see some general characteristics of this intruder and ways to approach it with a cautious friendliness.

Besides the minor bruises of life, my most intense experiences with pain have been three. I've lived since my teen years with a physical handicap, a severe curvature in my lower back. One "expert" graded it a seven on a scale of one to four. On seeing my X rays, most physicians express amazement that I'm still walking around and carrying on a normal life.

At the same time, my curvature doesn't show visibly. So, for better or for worse, I'm expected to live and function like a non-handicapped person. I'm constantly in situations that feel too difficult for me, but this is where life puts me.

My second intense experience with pain is that I've suffered deeply from the confusion of being a woman who didn't fit the mold for women. I didn't want to settle down and have children, I wanted to spend my life helping solve the problems of our human community and alleviating suffering. All the cultural forces of my life pushed me toward the mold of "good wife," "good mother." Although I love my children and husband, I still always feel the pain that I've spent my life's energy doing work I was not called to do.

I know I'm not the only person in the world who has experienced this. Many people have had their lives taken out of their hands, their dreams put aside, their gifts unsupported by a society that has other ideas for them. But knowing that others suffer the same never eases our own suffering, it only opens our heart to feel the pain of others as deeply as our own.

I've balanced as best I could all the strange elements, inward and outward, that I've been given to integrate in my life. As a helpmate and friend I had the loving support of a fine man. For twenty years we loved and wrangled and worked and played together. Then came my third intense experience with pain: at the age of forty-two, my dear husband, Tom Dix, died unexpectedly of a heart attack while sleeping beside me. Shortly after his death, all the pain of my life and my sympathy for others broke out into the writing of this book.

Although I have suffered pain, there are many kinds of terrible suffering I have not experienced. In some meditations here I have tried to empathize and search for what might be the gift in others' pain. But in the end, each of us must find and receive the particular gift in his or her own pain.

In these meditations is a hypothesis: *pain is not empty and meaningless: all pain has a gift at its core.* Even if someone else chose to be an instrument of pain for us, still, part of the cause of pain is a goal: the expansion of our own lives, a special newness, a gift for us. Similarly, if we're blaming ourselves for not following guidance or common sense, still there is also the hidden presence of a life force that pushed us awkwardly and instinctively toward a gift of growth. The immediate cause, the blame, and the source of the cure, the healing, for any particular pain—for these questions we must each find our particular answers. But pain is always an opportunity to grow in spirit: this part of the nature of pain must always be considered when we analyze our situation.

A goal can be one of the causes. If our growth is part of the purpose of pain, then the cure must include our willingness to grow. In pain, we are the egg cracking open for new and greater life, and we are the new and greater life itself struggling to be born. To grow in spirit is to grow in power and to be more, not less. Whatever has happened to us can make us more, bigger, greater.

Pain offers each of us a gift. The cost of our suffering can be recovered by looking for the gift and accepting it. Self-destructive bitterness fades when we accept the gift, the gift that comes in an ugly wrapping.

I know you didn't open this book out of philosophical curiosity. You are here with me because you know pain. Take your time in reading this; don't expect to read it all in one sitting. Each subject is dealt with in two ways: in an essay in which we can objectively "think about" an aspect of pain, and in a poetic meditation in which we step into the thought and see how it fits when we wear it. The personal application is important: "thinking about" life should not be a way to avoid living.

A great variety of thoughts about pain arise here, but they're all united by the theme that the purpose of pain is to bring gifts. A good idea might be to keep a pencil in your hand: as you read, allow yourself to write freely about your own pain. If you don't understand an essay or meditation, re-read, or just live with the thought for awhile, sleep on it. Or move on and come back. Find the diamond you are here to find, the clue to your particular pain. Let Love lead you through to the very last page and you will find your heart renewed and lightened.

May this the fruit of my life be a vehicle to help you receive the love and gifts that Grace is offering you.

MARTI MATTHEWS
Earlham School of Religion
May 30, 1989

I

*Pain Introduces Me
to the Other*

I

The "New" Comes

My life hasn't gotten bad enough yet for me to begin my real life.

—TOM FORSYTHE

ONE SUMMER AT THE INDIANA FIDDLERS' FEST WHERE WE were camping, I noticed in the crowd a young woman who dragged her feet slightly. I noticed her particularly because I have, as she seemed to have, the problem of a "barely visible" handicap. I seldom meet anyone who might understand the unique problems of almost-invisible handicaps.

Later I noticed that she was camping alone, and I went to talk with her. She was quiet, gentle, and cheerful, and she told me of new things she was trying to start in her life. She mentioned her problems with her feet and that the night before she had mustered the courage to try to do barn dancing. This brought me the opportunity to ask about her handicap.

In a simple manner she told me how her marriage had been unhappy, but she had resisted ending it. Finally, one day she jumped off a bridge onto an interstate expressway. She landed on her heels, and this was why she had trouble walking.

3

I was silenced, a little stunned. One doesn't do something that dangerous just to get attention; she must have truly intended to kill herself. It was sad that she had had to sink so far before she could change. She had resisted change to the edge of death. But Mercy had sent her back to try one more time; she finally let change happen, and then her life energy could once again flow constructively.

Sometimes there's no other way. We can watch our loved ones suffering, but we cannot change them: only they can do it. The wisest course may be to hold ourselves back and let our loved ones sink to the bottom before they reach the point of accepting change. And sometimes when our own pain gets worse it's because we are resisting change.

How long will we resist the new that wants to come?

How bad must it get?

It is important not to want pain. We should not glorify pain. Pain does not "please God," because The Source of Our Life is surely not sadistic. Pain is a warning system; if we glorify it rather than listen to it, harm will come to us.

Nor should we try to escape pain by seeking comfort before we've heard the warning. The only true escape from pain is to listen to it and respond to its instructions.

Pain is often a shell that we create. We try to keep a distance between pain and ourselves, to hold it out there at bay, hoping we might not have to feel it. As we hold it away from us, it begins to harden around us until we can feel less and less of ourselves or of anything at all.

But inside, the urge to grow is relentless. The only way to break this shell is to embrace our pain, to stop running from it and just experience what it feels like. When we stop sepa-

4

rating ourselves from it, we are open and newborn and ready for our first step in a new life.

Among people who were close to the earth, who observed the real nature of the other beings around them, the snake was a sacred symbol. The snake grows by completely shedding its old skin: it crawls out of the old and leaves it behind as it is born anew, fresh and vulnerable. The snake was the symbol of new life, and of life beyond death—the eternalness of the spirit.

We adult humans usually grow slowly; we hardly notice ourselves changing. But little changes build. At some point we discover we've outgrown our patterns. Like the snake, we discover that something in our exterior ways must change, shatter, crack open, and be shed, because something new inside needs room.

Part of us is comfortable with old ways, but part of us is not. Inside of us a battle goes on: we are the old and we are the new. Which part of us will win? The day of the new will always come; we can put it off, we can even think we've killed for good this threatening impulse. But nothing kills the urge to grow. If the energy to change is not yet strong enough, we will suffer on until our desire to change is sufficient to over- throw the old.

5

Pain is the shell that wants to be broken,
the skin that's too tight
   that wants to be shed.
Inside I'm crying,
   "Let me out!
   Let me out!
   Let me out!"

My pain is a womb that feels too full:
push, push, I must push,
I'm giving birth
to something new.
It hurts to push;
It hurts not to push.
I have no choice—
Something wants to come,
and it must.
I yell and cry,
I sweat and pant,
"Come forth, come forth!"
I try to relax and let it come.
My pain commands me:
bring the new forth
or die.

The New will come.
Pain is the challenge-cry of the young bull elk
to the old bull elk.
Is the old still king?
Will he reign another year

to sow his seed and breed what he breeds?—
seed perhaps too old to breed good life. . . .

Or is the new desire strong enough
to overthrow the old ways?
If the old wins again,
then pain must intensify
to strengthen the new.

Pain is the pathmaker for Change.
The New will come,
either today or tomorrow.

2

The Ruthless Force

There's a famous story about six blind men trying to describe an elephant. One feels a leg and says an elephant is big and round; another feels the tail and says an elephant is small and thin, and so on. I think we all describe God like that, depending on our own experiences. But I think the person who really knows what God is like is the seventh person—the one the elephant stomped on.
—ANNETTE REYNOLDS

WHEN WE ARE IN GREAT PAIN, PHYSICAL OR EMO-tional, we feel that we are up against a great impersonal force. Some people may call that force "God," but it doesn't feel like the God we thought we knew, the God in whom we want to believe. It feels closer to the old notion of Fate.

This force is gigantic. We can yell and scream, but it doesn't move. It doesn't seem to care how unbearable our suffering is. It doesn't respond to our pleading, although it has us on our knees. It's the silent steel eye of the tornado, the mocking heart of the gale, which smash and break apart without respect for emotion. It's the prairie fire that wipes the prairie clean so that new life can be born.

Pain brings us back to the present moment. As we stand here in pain, we find ourselves asking questions larger than "What happened yesterday?" and "What's going to happen tomorrow?" The before and after, the why and wherefore of life itself now come before our vision.

Is the force of pain a face of Love? This we do not know yet. But surprisingly, pain places us in the midst of love. Once we have known great pain, our hard hearts are cracked open, and we realize the secret everyone holds inside: we are all in pain. Pain humbles and levels us all until we are finally equals; we are finally bonded in love through compassion. It was said well by the philosopher Gabriel Marcel: "In the realm of mystery there are no generalized solutions, only communion, testimony and witness."[1] We are all waiting with the same questions, trying in our bewildered ways to understand the Ruthless Force that we have encountered in our suffering.

Pain is the stark presence
  of unfathomable and ultimate mystery,
the endless dark and confusing forest,
the skulking presence of danger.

It is the mouth of the large and frightening ocean
waiting for our exhaustion,
the hurricane tossing us in chaos.

Pain is the existential encounter with the Before and After,
which we cannot remember or imagine.
The Force.
The Great Force.
We do not remember how to command it to obey—
if we ever knew.
It gives no warning,
It shows no mercy to the tired and weak.
It silences logic
  and evades analysis.
It speaks only one word: *"Listen!*
Listen to me. Pay attention to me."
Reluctantly, all our energies are pulled into a single focus:
the unknown that has brought us pain.

Pain breaks the proud,
  quiets the haughty.
    It levels all people.
All equally wait in silence for pain to reveal its message.

3

Pain Raises Questions

*Thought is born of failure. . . .To think is to confess a lack
of adjustment which we must stop to consider.*
                                            —L.L. WHYTE

IN MANY SOCIETIES ADOLESCENTS ARE BROUGHT INTO
adulthood through the gates of pain. We shiver when we read
about the initiation rites for some young people; we would
never do these things to our children. We protect them from
pain as long as we can, just as we protect ourselves. Comfort
is one of our gods.

But consequently, our children stay children for an amazingly long time. It's easy to identify the twenty-five-year-old
children in our society. Probably by the time they've reached
thirty they've been initiated by accident: they've been in and
out of jail or emergency rooms, or they've been to war; they've
lost jobs, created new life out of wedlock, or already known
the pain of love-marriage-divorce.

We shrink from this reality: it is pain that carries us across
the river into adulthood.

11

Helen Keller tells of an awful time of shame she experienced when she was twelve. The strangest circumstances made it appear that she had plagiarized a story to get the favor of her school principal. She was cruelly interrogated by eight teachers. The blind and deaf child had to face them alone, without her beloved Annie Sullivan beside her. Helen didn't look back and laugh at the pain; it was a terrible thing to go through, and she still felt sympathy for herself when she remembered it later. But she observed that while before this incident she had been a child, the painful event had given her self-awareness. "Gradually I emerged from the penumbra of that experience with a mind made clearer by trial and with a truer knowledge of life."[2]

All through our creative years we feel the power of being human, as if there's nothing so great as our accomplishments. Pain stops us; like a great train signal arm, it says, "Go no further. Look in all directions. There are limits to your power. You are not the center of the universe! Despite your anger and fury, you cannot will the pain away."

Who is it that has taken control of our lives, and what is it up to? God, Nature, Pain, Fate, the Universe, Destiny, Karma? Whatever it is, will it respond, will it move? Why is it allowing this to happen? Often our churches and parents and teachers have given us answers to these questions before they've allowed us to ask them. Perhaps the stories of our sacred books and great literature are important not so much for their answers as for the questions they try to address. After experiencing pain, we are finally brought to the beginning of responsible humanness: we are asking the questions that lead to conscious living.

It may take us a long time to find our own answers to the questions. In the meantime, we cannot avoid relating to this Power that confronts us. We will have to make a choice: to believe, in spite of all, that the Greater Power (the "Other") is trustable and therefore we can go with the flow of wherever life is carrying us, or we can try to fight this other force to the end. Either choice is all right, but one makes for a harder life than the other.

Sometimes we secretly enjoy fighting and suffering, feeling that we're heroes standing against Fate. Richard Moss described poignantly our love for drama, even when fighting isn't getting us out of our suffering: "There's so much more emotional drama, more sense of 'me,' in fighting against life than there is in yielding to life and becoming life's lover."[3] Why not try an experiment: Try relaxing and see where this ferocious determined Other is taking us. Where does this road lead, where is this river trying to go? Why do we fear it? What have we to lose by leaning *into* the experience? We can fight against what's happening to us, or we can take the same energy and throw ourselves into the experience. Perhaps when we've suffered enough we'll try relaxing into life instead of fighting against it.

Pain tells me that my life is not my own.
I thought I was sole owner of this vehicle,
but I find a mysterious hidden Other
directing me this way and that,
away from what I'm reaching for
and toward that which I choose not.
Another is dragging me down a dark road:
how long is this road?
Where does it go?
Why must I go down here?
the Other knows but doesn't tell me.
Is it kind or is it cruel,
this Other who has taken control of my life?
What does it want with me?
My will is helpless.
My only choice is to cooperate with the Other,
or die fighting.

4

Pain Tames and Reconnects Us

. . . the idea of sacrifice consists mainly in the acceptance by the isolated personality of transpersonal goals and alignment with transpersonal Nature, rather than fighting for the self-centered personality itself.
—ALYCE GREENE AND ELMER GREENE

I HAVE A QUESTION: WHY DO I HAVE A CROOKED BACK?

I mean, I want to know the *real why*, not the little *why* that physicians and scientists give. They still leave me with the big questions that really matter: Why me? Why all of us? Why this?

There is a metaphor about pain that speaks to my heart; it is an answer for the "Why me?" and "Why this?" Perhaps others will relate to this image. It's the notion of "being tamed." I keep feeling that my crooked back is for me like reins on a horse, and some Force larger than I am wants to be part of my life.

There is a scene in the movie "Man from Snowy River" in which ranch hands are chasing after a herd of wild horses, trying to recapture a runaway stallion. The cowboys are cunning in their pursuit until they think they will have the wild horses trapped at a precipice. The horses run at full speed toward the edge, the cowboys riding expectantly behind. The wild horses arrive at the edge and, without hesitating, continue on right over the cliff.

The cliff is actually not a cliff but an acute dropoff; the stone angles downward at an extremely sharp drop, but the wild horses are able to keep their footing on its surface. The cowboys arrive at the edge; they cannot pursue the wild horses because their own mounts won't follow. But the man from Snowy River and his horse do not hesitate: they, too, go right over the edge and disappear. At the bottom it's possible for the man to trap the wild herd and maneuver it back, and the escaped stallion is recaptured.

How could a tamed horse follow the wild horses? Was the horse of the man from Snowy River truly tame? What we think of as "taming" is that the horse must lose its wild, free nature. If the man's horse had lost its beautiful wild nature, it would not have pursued the wild horses over the edge. This horse had accepted running with the man, but the horse and the man had become one—sometimes the man led, and sometimes the horse led. All the strength and wisdom of each was at the disposal of the other. Together they could accomplish things that neither could accomplish alone.

To us, being brought to live in community with others and with the Other can feel like "sacrifice" or pain. We feel that finding and accepting our useful place in a larger group forces us to give up something of our own will.

16

But what we gain from living with others is meaning. Only the community, besides giving us others' help and wisdom, can also give meaning and importance to our gifts and specialness. It is through our sharing that we become beloved. Love is our reward. Meaning is our participation in the creation of the world. It is a relational activity: ourselves with others and the Other, all putting forth our efforts to bring life to an increase.

We can exist without meaning, we can just experience the joy of being, as do flowers and trees that no one sees, or wild horses running for their own joy. But the human question "Why am I alive?" can be answered only by living in community.

I am a wild horse, and Someone is trying to tame me.
I have my own direction,
running free with the wind,
but an Other imposes its will against me.
I am led in circles and patterns and routines,
cramped, constrained, confined,
sometimes struck with sharp pain.
I want to run wild
according to my own strong will.
The Other says I'm being "trained";
I must learn to serve.
The Other has intentions I don't understand:
"We will harness your power;
you will be both beautiful and useful."

All a wild horse knows is the joy of living,
running free and independently.
Who has a claim to my life besides me?
This "trainer" talks about others whom I can help
when we "harness my power."
"Am I a slave now?" I ask.
The Other says I can be free again
when I learn to obey Wisdom.
This is a new kind of freedom to me—
to be free through obedience.
Wild horses know nothing of this.
All of my mind and body rebel,
but pain is wearing me down.
Perhaps I must consider "freedom through obedience"
    and "usefulness."

What's in it for me?
The Other says people will "love" me
when my power and beauty are harnessed to help them.
Wild horses want nothing from others;
we want to be independent and free,
"enjoying" until we die.
Why should I want this "love"?—
    maybe it will hurt, too.
But pain strikes me again:
perhaps "love" will feel better.

I already see that I'm not alone;
the presence of the Other tells me
that my separateness
was an illusion.

5

Death Speaks

Your life feels different on you, once you greet death and understand your heart's position. You wear your life like a garment from the mission bundle sale ever after—lightly because you realize you never paid nothing for it, cherishing because you know you won't ever come by such a bargain again.

—LOUISE ERDRICH

AFTER MY HUSBAND DIED I OFTEN WATCHED WITH WONder the pairs of ducks floating on a nearby pond. What do they experience when their mates die? I wondered. What came to me was this: they experience surprise, confusion, and the same sense of great loss that we feel. But they do not experience the fear and sense of "tragedy" that we experience; they place no value judgements on the disappearance of their mates. They must adapt themselves as we must, but they don't fear the event as threatening the solidity of existence.

Animals and plants (as far as we can tell) accept the parameters of the game: they create what they are able to create, and

20

they learn what they are born to learn. It seems that only humans fight against the natural structure. "Regarding the migration of the eels," says Neils Bohr, Nobel Prize winner in physics, "it is just because they do not know where they are going that they always do it perfectly." Only humans must make a choice to work with nature or fight against it.

Animals and plants truly "live in grace," and humans "fall" by the overexertion of will and ego. We force and control all we can until pain teaches us humility, our limits; pain reminds us that there is a much larger story going on than the one of our little selves, and there are greater powers we must respect. We are not nothing, but we are not All-That-Is, either.

Walking through the mysteries of life is like walking anywhere in the darkness. The ground is there beneath our feet: solid, sure, it's really there. We feel unsure of ourselves only because we're accustomed to "seeing" our way with our physical eyes, and to seeing ahead, beyond where we're standing. When we approach death, we cannot see ahead with our physical eyes. But we will feel neither more nor less safe at this moment than we've figured out how to feel throughout our lives.

While we are living we can learn to be aware of and comfortable with all the mystery that we live in. We can become accustomed not only to the physical world but to the before and after that surrounds it, and to unseen energy as well as the seen and controllable. Perhaps Neils Bohr was wrong: perhaps the eels *do* know where they're going, but not in the conscious, anaylytical way that we call "knowing." Instincts and intuitions are, in fact, ways of knowing. Perhaps we "know" where we're going after death just as surely as the eels know where they're going.

It behooves us to expand our awareness beyond our physical limits. When we stop running from mysteries and relax and trust the world as it's been given, then we can start to live in this world with full power. If we trust what we know beyond what our analytical minds know, then even death may not need to be so frightening.

We cannot live fully, creatively, healthily, peacefully, until we've found a way to accept death, because if death isn't solid, then life isn't solid. Pain loses its power to intimidate us when we come again to trust the processes of this reality: we "pass through" and grow and create and "pass on," and this process is safe.

One of the most precious gifts I've received from the death of my husband is the gift of "My Own Death." I know with a vivid awareness that I will die. I could die tomorrow. Tom was young, he was involved in "very important work," he was "needed," and he was careful and wise, and none of this stopped death from carrying him on.

Awareness of our own death enables us to live more fully. We become efficient—we stop playing around in trivia and get down to the main substance of life: given limited time, what do I *most* want to do? What is my greatest gift—that which comes from my unique experiences, that which the world wants to receive from me before I die? Let me do it! Soon I will pass on, as did my loved ones and every life on earth before me. Passing on is safe and solid. But while I am here let me give my *best* contribution.

The sun comes up and goes down.
The ducks float, their mates die,
they're confused and in pain for a while,
then they go on floating.
The hungry cat pursues the mouse,
eats it, rests, and pursues no more.
The mouse feels fright for a moment
but gives itself to something larger,
then passes on.
The hungry rabbit finds no food
and burrows down and dies;
it doesn't cry, it simply leaves.
The world does not ask why.
Why do I?
My grandmother died,
and my great-grandmother, too.
They stepped forth among us from "nowhere"
and lived and learned and "died."
And *I will die too.*
I am only passing through,
learning while I travel.
Like a plant, my life consists of feeling and growing.
Like a fish, I'm born into a "school,"
I swim through my world seeing many things.
Like an animal, I grow by moving
    across a terrain of experience.
My pain reminds me
that the world that seems so real
is transitory and illusory;
there are Hidden Forces that bring us and take us. . . .

II

Grace, and the Nature of Pain

6

There Is Hope

You do not have to fight to trust the thrust of your own life. That thrust is always meant to lead you toward your own best fulfillment. . . .

—SETH

A BEAUTIFUL, DEEP, FRESHWATER SPRING IN PONCE DE-Leon State Park, DeLand, Florida, connects to a larger lake by means of a little dam. A small opening beneath the dam allows divers to swim from the spring to the lake. Divers like to explore the depths of the spring and then find the tunnel that leads to the opening. But the sediment on the spring bottom is very fine; sometimes, when divers get into the tunnel, the sediment is stirred up by their swimming, and they become disoriented. They try to turn back and flail in circles, stirring up more sediment until they can no longer tell which direction is up and which is forward. Many times the fire department is called to send someone down into the little tunnel and pull out the body of a diver who was unable to find the opening into the lake.

27

Many times I've thought of that frightening situation—to be close to the end of your breath, to know there is an opening somewhere, to grope for it, but to panic and only stir up the chaos and danger more. The diver who can stay calm, knowing confidently that there is an opening, and move directly toward it by instinct will arrive at the open lake. The diver is lost who panics and fails to continue toward the opening but tries to circle back. There is a point of no return in that tunnel; one must go through the door and go through it calmly.

Pain is similar. We feel we are drowning in chaos, grief, emotion, burden, strain; the situation is impossible, unbearable. There seems no way out. The way out, however, is often obvious to an outside observer but unacceptable to the person in pain. It's the last door on earth the person wants to take.

You may try to share what you see with a friend in pain:

"It seems to me the only way out of your pain is:

to stop caring about this person who broke your heart.
to stop caring about what other people think.
to stop fighting what your body is doing.
to exercise and eat right.
to stop drinking, smoking.
to stand up for yourself.
to forgive.
to learn to be happy alone."

What will your friend most likely say?
"I can't."

Do we also do this? Do we know the door out of our pain but refuse to take it?

* * *

The way gets narrower and narrower. There is some way my deepest self wants to grow. "I," my conscious ego-self, am refusing to move into this new and open place, but my soul is determined that I will. My choices are getting fewer and fewer. Like the diver, I try to go back, try to stay my old familiar self in my comfortable ways, but something won't let me. The pressure from both within and without is greater and greater. I continue to say,

"I can't." (I don't want to have to. . . .)

"I don't know what to do." (I don't want to do it. . . .)

There is hope; there is a way out. Panic, tightness, worry, fury, fear—these are our defenses against our salvation. Although it may seem ironic and illogical, the truth may be that doing less, staying still, *relaxing*, quieting our thoughts, may enable us to find the safe way. Then we must freely choose to go through the door, to not resist the growth that our Life Force desires.

Pain is the face of a coin,
and on the underside is Hope.
Pain tells me this only seems like hell:
As long as I feel pain
I know I'm not dead;
things could still be changed.

Here in almost-hell
I feel I'm suffocating, drowning,
groping desperately in the dark water.
Pain points to the way out.
It says, "There *is* a door!
I'm guiding you; don't fight me."
Pain is my friend
who wants to guide me toward the light
when I want to go on
walking in the darkness,
the friend who wants to speak
when I want only to hear myself.
Pain tells me to relax,
   to open to the unacceptable;
then I'll see the doorway
   out of almost-hell.

7

Grace Tames Pain

As swimmers dare to lie face to the sky
and waters bear them,
as hawks rest upon air
and air sustains them,
so would I learn to attain
freefall, and float
into Creator Spirit's deep embrace,
knowing no effort earns
that all-surrounding grace.

—DENISE LEVERTOV

GRACE IS THE GENTLE PRESENCE OF DIVINE LOVE AL-
ways with us, upholding us, but not demanding our attention
in the manner of pain. Pain is more visible than Grace.

At some point I started what I called my "miracle box." In
it I record the daily "miracles" that happen to me and to
friends—the events that some write off as "luck" or "coinci-
dence." These events are as much hard evidence and scientific
data as anything else that happens.

I saw myself drawing large conclusions about "life" when

31

things went against me, but when things went for me I would write them off as "mere chance." Every day, besides having puzzling and negative experiences, I was experiencing positive evidence that I am upheld. Both are data to be remembered equally. So when my faith-that-I-am-upheld weakens, I go back to my miracle box and review the evidence.

Perhaps I shouldn't use the word "miracle." A Quaker friend, Richard Boyajian, says: "I can't use the word 'miraculous,' for that implies a supernatural event, and my belief is that supernatural events are impossible. If it can happen, it's natural."[1]

We can take a negative path through life and dig ourselves into a hole, where we can't see above the rim and where all looks bleak. I have focused on the positive and found it solid; it gives greater and greater life. Life does uphold us, if we don't fight it!

The loving Power that will carry us safely from the beginning of our story to the end—this I have called Grace. Grace will help us handle pain. The Source of Our Life does not abandon us but, like a mother, will be with us always to help us grow and become all that we can be. We will have guidance and strength sufficient to receive whatever gifts our pain is trying to give us.

Does Pain come alone?
Some say yes and some say no.
The nays say it comes with its twin:
Pain, the very visible guide,
Grace, the unseen merciful guide.

Pain, the bold unwanted guide;
Grace, waiting to be sought for and asked.

Pain, the commanding taskmaster;
Grace, the alert parent
   there to catch us when we fall.

Pain, whose shadow, fear,
    beckons us to drown in the depths;
Grace, whose loving arms
    uphold the trusting spirit.

Grace the Illuminator
    for those who ask humbly
    and wait patiently
    and listen openly.

Grace the merciful with her shadow, Time:
    together they heal and strengthen.
To those who perceive their presence
they bring the balms of
    sufficient strength,
    intuitive understanding,
    patient growth.

33

For those who ask,
Grace tames Pain.
First she takes the power from the shadow, fear:
She breaks the center of the fearful storm.
She weakens the grip on the tightening body:
She breathes confidence into any lungs that breathe
   her air.
Grace smiles warmly on the hurting heart and body;
when Grace is allowed in,
Pain's frown can relax.

Pain the driving force,
Grace the gentle guide:
the creative twins
Who couple and give birth to Growth,
the Divine Force that beckons us to be more.
We, the created, humbly bow and say
"So be it."

8

Saying the Question

Ask, and you will receive; seek, and you
will find; knock, and the door will be opened. . . .
— JESUS OF NAZARETH

IT IS VERY IMPORTANT TO SAY CLEARLY WHAT WE WANT. When we bring ourselves to say out loud, "I have a problem; it's X; I want to solve this; I could use some help," then we have the physical sensation that we're suddenly standing on a path, we're *on* the path, it's under our feet. We still don't know the solution, but saying the question seems to start our movement in a direction.

I have a prayer for these situations; I call it my "Help!" prayer. It goes "Help! Help, help, help, help!" (Obviously, repeatable.)

One of my first important encounters with Grace came through marrying a mathematician. (I remember sitting in my high school geometry class and wondering, "What kind of a woman would marry a mathematician?") The religion of my childhood had emphasized the "nobility of suffering": we are

35

so sinful we deserve to suffer; we can earn eternal rewards by suffering; we prove how strong we are by suffering; we can purify ourselves by hurting ourselves; and God will know how much we love him when we suffer in his name.

My husband, Tom, did not believe in this theology. We never discussed it in terms of religious beliefs, but to a mathematician all problems are solvable; that's why we have brains! If I complained about something, he would brainstorm on what could be done. I would explain why the problem was necessary and why we had to live with it, but he would insist on solving it. I gradually came to realize that many problems are solvable and that we don't have to suffer as much as I had thought. Nor did it feel sinful or contrary to nature to solve problems and be happy. As my beliefs changed, I, too, took to putting my mind in gear to solve what I could.

I'm aware that not all problems are solvable by analysis and that not all pain can be made to disappear easily. Fortunately, we have not only a rational brain but also an intuitive brain, through which we are connected to wisdom larger than ourselves.

The direction of analytical thinking is toward focus, concentrated effort, attack. The direction of intuitive thinking is towards openness, connectedness, receptivity. Both have their value, and they complement each other. But when analysis has failed to solve the problem, where can we turn for a solution except toward something bigger than ourselves? In my experience, this idea proves true:

> In normal living and in day-by-day experience, all the knowledge you need is available. You must, however, believe that it is, put yourself in a position to receive it by looking inward and remaining open to your intuitions, and most important, by *desiring* to receive it.
>
> —SETH[2]

When we state our desire to receive help or guidance we open a door and invite inside the sources that Life has waiting to help us. I'm amazed at how many times I've asked a clear question before I fell asleep at night, asked although unclear of whom I was asking, and then have had a dream that answered my question. Our lives seem not to be islands; we are surrounded by help and concern, although we know not the why or the source.

After my husband died I was worried about our financial future until I had an amusing and vivid dream that restored my confidence. I dreamed that an airplane flew over my back yard while I was outside and that a member of the Mafia was on that plane with a suitcase full of money. The plane suddenly had a terrible problem and was partly torn open; it looked as though it would crash. So the man threw the suitcase out of the plane, and it landed in my back yard (of course). The story went on with further details. After pondering the various interpretations I could give it, what felt right to me was that there are more ways under heaven then I've begun to imagine that the universe could help me if I needed it! It isn't only up to me: if I try my best I will be supported and helped, and in ways I might never imagine. When we commit ourselves, our commitment attracts commitment from the loving Source of Life.

Try it! Try asking a question or asking for help, addressing yourself to whomever you want—the Universe, God, one's higher self, or just "anybody out there." Then be open and aware for a few days. The answer will come, in one form or another: while waking or sleeping, through the words of a friend or foe, through a fleeting thought or a large event. These are not coincidences, these are responses: Life will respond when we commit ourselves to finding solutions.

I am looking and looking for the key
that will enable me
to get on top of my pain.
I want to control the situation.
When I realize that I have a choice—
that I can live with pain
or I can find the way out of it—
then the way begins to open.

When I turn my pain into a question,
the question is a calling out to Grace.
The merciful Mother begins to come toward me;
I sense her presence faintly.
She calls the answer to me from afar.
I hear it vaguely;
I hear the first line of her instructions.
With my ears now alert,
I hear more.
Very suddenly we are one!
The Gentle Guide within
mercifully leads me to understand my pain.
When I humble myself to ask for help,
Grace, the Merciful Mother, brings me to the place
    of peace.
I am never alone with Pain.

9

Learning to See in Fog

The body and mind together do present a united, self-regulating, healing, self-clearing system. Within it, each problem contains its own solution if it is honestly faced. Each symptom, mental or physical, is a clue to the resolution of the conflict behind it, and contains within it the seeds of its own healing.

—SETH

THE DESIRE OF NATURE IS GROWTH, HEALTH, BALANCE, peace, joy, fruitfulness. Pain is a feedback system within nature. It draws attention to some particular part of life where we are ready to grow and expand. If we cannot understand clearly the direction our pain is trying to suggest, we needn't worry: if we don't understand the first time, pain will repeat itself and will speak louder each time. Some theme will repeat over and over in our lives; again and again we face the same issue. We think we've solved this, but then once more the same old problem pops up like a shadowy stalker, unpredictably ruining things. When something in us wants to expand and heal, that part of us will create disaster after disaster to bring our conscious attention to this broken place where there's an opening for our expansion. Sooner or later we'll get the message; something will gradually become clear.

We may feel hounded and ask what is stalking us and why. The best approach is to turn our attention toward it without judgement; we just want to see its face.

Don't try to oppose or control what assaults you. Don't label it as good or bad. Don't try to stop the natural processes; just wait with patience, and observe.

We embrace our stalker because we want to heal this terrible hurt. "What are you trying to say?" we might ask. "And what would make you feel better? Where are you hiding—in my guts? In my feet? Are you choking my throat? Are you lashing out at others with my arms, trying to protect me? To protect me from what?" We should speak lovingly to this part of ourselves that cares about us. Our pain is the beggar within us, begging for a response to our own unseen need.

In trying to uncover the source of our pain we might look into the messages we were given in the past, hurtful beliefs that someone taught us long ago and that we may be repeating to ourselves:

"I'm always. . . ." "I never. . . ." "I can't. . . ."
"I must/I have to/there is no choice. . . ."
"I need/I must have. . . ."
"Life is. . . ."

These messages could be the source of our pain. When we say to ourselves the opposite ideas, do our bodies feel healthier and more relaxed? Do our emotions feel healthier?

As we don't resist our hidden pain but watch it and feel it without judgement, without fear, the paralyzing grip is broken. We can breathe again and think. When we stop running and just feel what we're feeling, we allow some space for our strength to catch up. Stephen Levine tells how he found himself with a terrible fear but stuck in there and didn't run from his feelings until he had loosened their grip. He describes his struggle:

> Staying with the investigation of this pain and resistance—the tension in the body, the fever in the mind—just taking a breath at a time, there began to arise a little space around these images. Slowly they began to float in a choiceless awareness. As I allowed the resistance to just be there as an object of investigation, the pain began to melt in the mind, the fever broke. The resistance began to dissolve. And at last awareness had direct access to the images themselves, no longer hindered by an unexplored fearfulness and sense of helplessness within.[3]

Impatience and fear may be our enemies in understanding our pain. Self-knowledge comes to us in layers, as we are strong enough to peel it away. Courage and persistance and patience will win eventually.

Pain has many faces.
It's a friend who jumps from form to form,
the gradually-changing amoeba,
the untouchable ghost who taunts us,
the weed we thought had been cleared from our garden.
It's the Mr. Hyde of Dr. Jekyll—
the hidden side of a bright life.
Pain cries out against these splits;
it reaches out to pull together
that which has been apart.
It does not want to be Mr. Hyde,
but first it must clearly be Mr. Hyde
so that we can see our alienated part
and welcome it home again.
Pain is the mirror
in which we see invisible parts of ourselves:
our choices, our values,
our negligence, our weaknesses,
our ideas, our beliefs.
Our thoughts live in our body
and in the emotions we experience.
Pain tries to show us: "these are the thoughts you
   are thinking,
and this is the path you're on."

We want to see—
And we don't want to see.
Pain may be the firm friend or the committed enemy,
the hot love or the icy hate,

but never the indifferent shrug,
never the lukewarm passing.
What is unimportant to us cannot cause us pain.
What am I caring about?
My pain could end if I stopped caring.
Perhaps I'll choose to stop soon;
perhaps I'll never choose to stop.

When I look into the mirror with my eyes open,
when I embrace myself as I am,
Love enables me to see where I'm going.
With my eyes open to see
And my heart open to be guided,
Whatever path I'm on is safe.

10

Pain Speaks

The more we don't wait properly, the longer it takes.
—Friends Journal

MODERN PEOPLE IN GENERAL ARE NOT SENSITIVE LIS-
teners. We attack our problems by throwing gross energy at
them, like elephants trying to move all by force. Nor are we
objective observers: we cling to a belief in the omnipotence
of our own doing and thinking—surely we can handle any
problem by throwing more time or money at it or by cutting
it out by force.

We believe we don't need to listen to the source of the
trouble. If people behave badly we lock them away or execute
them. If a group of people is troublesome, send in the Guard.
As drugs and crime increase, we increase our police force.
Unfortunately, the source of the drug problem is not the sup-
pliers but the demanders, and we don't want to deal patiently
with the complex original problem. But solutions of force
never stop trouble at its source, so the problem keeps coming
back in bigger amounts. How much easier life could be if we

listened carefully and with openness to find the root causes of problems.

Did the Europeans when first arriving here have this current American tendency to try to conquer all problems with force? We are told the first pilgrims arrived with a sense of gratefulness and cooperated with those already living here. They felt upheld by life and believed that the opportunity to solve their problems in this new land was a gift.

But quickly the enthusiasm developed into a spirit of "conquer the gift" and grab all you can for yourself. The Native American way of life based on cooperation with the gifts around us was written off as "primitive." To the Europeans, people anywhere in the world who did not "conquer" nature were inferior, because nature itself was not trusted. We come from a belief system that says that the life force is our enemy, that there is nothing to trust but our own selves and our own doing, so we throw our elephant force frantically against every problem.

Pain is a gift of nature; it is the voice of a guide helping us grow into mature beings. But our American-ness may be a hindrance in dealing with our personal pain. We will want to conquer the problem with a quick and easy solution—pills, surgery, divorce, a cocktail, the lottery, moving out of the neighborhood, moving out of the house. And almost everyone around us will urge these solutions on us. But like our society, we'll find that the quick solution doesn't end the problem. Eventually we must listen to something. We must cooperate with nature, give up on forcing a way out of pain, and wait to discover the one way that will really work. Ram Dass put it this way: "Truth waits for laws unclouded by longing."

If we cannot wait properly, we'll find that pain has more force than we do. Pain is an awkward system—it has no respect for logic, or for notions like "keeping face" or "dignity." Its voice is actually quiet; but if we don't hear it when it speaks

45

gently, then pain can be crude and rough—it will just throw us against the wall and say "listen!" Eventually we will have to let go of our dignity and listen. Inside this apparent bully there is a gentle love trying to speak to us and lead us into growth.

One of our defenses against change is to keep talking to ourselves. What we say comes out of our past and upholds a way of life or a point of view that's familiar to us. But when the ways of the past seem insufficient to get rid of pain, then it's time to be open to hearing something new. This requires silencing our mind, shushing the words that have upheld the old ways. In the Castaneda story of a young man learning the ways of the Indians in northern Mexico, the old man advises Carlos in how to "stop the world," as he calls this silence that allows the new:

> Whenever the dialogue stops, the world collapses and extraordinary facets of ourselves surface, as though they had been kept heavily guarded by our words.[4]

If our current ideas were working, we would already be out of pain. There's something we haven't thought of yet. We must be ready for a surprise. Although the way out may be something we don't want to hear, if we are truly ready to be free of pain we must be quiet and listen. As Elspeth Huxley puts it,

> If you fire off a question, it is like firing off a gun—bang it goes, and everything takes flight and runs for shelter. But if you sit quite still and pretend not to be looking, all the little facts will come and peck round your feet, situations will venture forth from thickets, and intentions will creep out and sun themselves on a stone. . . .[5]

Pain shouts,
but in a language I don't understand.
I'm trying to get the message;
I'm trying for all I'm worth.
Maybe I'm trying too hard.

I sit perplexed . . . silent. . . .
A breeze caresses me like a cool blessing.
But it's not a breeze, it's a whisper!
Underneath the noise, the storm,
is a whisper;
I couldn't hear it
because I was trying so hard.
In a moment of stillness
I heard the voice that was always there.

When I am full of effort and thought
the size of pain must be big
to get my attention,
but the voice of pain is naturally quiet.
I must listen very carefully.
I must free myself of expectations,
of wishes,
of self-imposed limits
and old ideas that work no more.
I cannot hear
what I don't want to hear.
I must empty myself of my own noise
to hear a whisper.

II

Naming the Pain

You shall know the truth,
And the truth shall make you free.
                    —JESUS OF NAZARETH

THERE IS SOMETHING IMMENSELY HEALING ABOUT SAY-
ing one's truth. The problem that had been a vague and dark
cloud hanging over us takes form and size. We know what we
are dealing with, and we feel we've taken some command over
our lives.

In a course I took on sacraments, the class studied various
ways of experiencing symbolic expression of ideas. I was excited when we studied the fairy tale "Rumpelstiltskin." It was
about me! It stated a problem I had and so freed me from it.

The story of Rumpelstiltskin tells of a miller who bragged
that his daughter could spin straw into gold. Instead of standing up to him, she tries to do it. With the help of unexpected
force in the form of a strange little man, she manages to do
it twice, although the price is great. Finally, however, the price
is to be her own child; just as she has become a slave to an
unsolved problem, her child will also be controlled by it. She

48

is told that the only hope she has is to find out the name of whoever has been helping her do the impossible. She finally discovers his name and says it out loud—Rumpelstiltskin— and immediately it begins to lose its power and melt away. "The security of hell," says the devil in *Doctor Faustus,* "is not to be informed on, that it is protected from speech, that it cannot be made public. . . ."[6]

I remember a friend who, as an adult, asked a serious question of his adult brother, perhaps something about sex, or a similar important part of life that's little talked about. His brother's only response was "That question should never arise." But what cannot be talked about cannot be handled. It can then rule us, like the strange, contorted little Rumpelstilskin. When we put a problem into words we are bringing it into the light, where it can be examined; then it already begins to lose its control over us.

In our minds is an unrealistic ideal that makes us ashamed to admit we have problems, as if no one else in the world has them, as if we should be perfect. We will never be perfect, because we will always be growing. To see where we could grow is not a judgement on the way we've been; we have not been "bad." We've just outgrown our ways, as children outgrow their clothes. Our old ways worked before, but they hurt now and are feeling like a "problem." To say what we don't want in our lives is to declare ourselves its equal and our intention to be free.

Michael Crichton tells a story of camping in a tent in India when he heard terrible noises in the night; it sounded as if an elephant were outside his tent. For an hour he lay terrified in his bed. Finally, he could no longer stand the pressure of not knowing what it was, so he tiptoed to the tent window and looked out into the dark. Right at the window he saw this giant eye; yes, an elephant was outside his tent! So he went back to bed and slept soundly.

Later, he wondered why he'd been able to sleep soundly

after he knew he was truly in danger. He realized that not knowing the exact truth of the situation caused fear to grow into hysteria. Once he was sure of what he was dealing with, the fear could stop growing. "Subsequent emotions may not be pleasant, but the hysteria stops. . . .We feel we are afraid to look, when actually it is not-looking that makes us afraid. The minute we look, we cease being afraid."[7]

A friend of mine was in a promising but puzzling relationship with a person of the opposite gender. She told me she did not feel afraid as long as she was truthful, and she knew when she was being truthful because her heart was light. I was surprised; this sounded much like an ancient Egyptian story I'd heard of a boy who searched the world trying to learn how to make his heart as light as a feather. The reason he needed to learn this was because after death, the hearts of the dead were placed on the scale of truth and justice and weighed against a feather; if one's heart was lighter than the feather of truth, one passed the test of having lived right.

Saying the truth lightens our spirits because it makes us the equal of the unknown that often causes fear. The heavy fog lifts, and we find we are standing on firm ground. Truth is solid. It's also healthy; saying the truth heals. Standing on truth, we can begin taking from our pain the gift that it holds.

When I name my pain I begin to know it.
When I discover its name,
when I decide to stand up for myself
and say its name out loud—
"Rumpelstiltskin!"—
it begins to lose its power.

When I find the name of my pain
I can find the treatment it wants:

Frustration calls out for patience,

but despair cries for help from others.

Grief may want expression,

Loneliness calls for reaching out,

Confusion begs for discussion.

When I speak its name
I can wrestle with my pain as an equal.
I know my opponent.
I know its form and size.
Sometimes my pain will be on top
and for a moment pin me down.
But then I rise and handle it,
I am strong enough.
I *can* do what I must do.

I can do it.

I'm not afraid of you, Pain;

Whatever your name is,

mine is always courage.

51

12

The Cup of Blessings: Receiving Our Gifts

An empty cup is the most fillable.
—DAG HAMMERSKJÖLD

ONE DAY I WOKE UP AND FOUND MYSELF MARRIED AND raising little children, neither of which was what I had wanted to do with my life. This work was doubly hard because of the curvature of my lower back. Everything took more energy from me than from other people. If I had been physically stronger I could have tried to do what other strong women try: to raise children and have a career at the same time. But my physical limitations precluded that strenuous possibility.

I felt bitter. I loved my children and my husband, but my heart was always turned toward what I couldn't do.

In a discussion group, I was assigned to read a strange book that I would never have read on my own. In it the author declared that life is reincarnational, we live many lives, but in particular that we *choose* our lives. We chose to be who we are because this situation would offer us an opportunity to grow in a way that our souls wanted to grow. We chose our sex, our parents and siblings, our bodies, our time period in history, because all this would be a prime opportunity to accomplish something we wanted to do.

"You mean, I might have *chosen* to be a housewife raising kids and to have a crooked back?" I thought to myself incredulously. "Why would I want this?!"

I no sooner asked the question then the answer came. Just one week earlier at the end of a workshop I attended, we were asked to make a wish for the person with whom we were sharing. My partner made a strange wish for me. Using her own vocabulary, she said, "I hope that Marti may become the Buddha she is trying to become."

I had studied enough of Buddhism to understand what she was pointing to. In my words, it would be attaining wisdom—that is, understanding what life is all about and gaining the ability to live by solid principles.

So when I asked myself, "Why would I choose to be a housewife with a crooked back?" I suddenly realized what it was that I was doing with my life: gaining wisdom!

My crooked back was like reins on a horse for me. I knew that I have an enormous amount of energy and that without this restraint I would be highly successful at "something" in the ordinary world. My crooked back had directed that energy away from material and temporary success toward something eternal: wisdom.

And the situation of homemaking was perfect for "ruminating" about life. Each day my husband faced a demanding world with specific problems to think about. Raising children and managing a house was demanding and required intelligence, but with a broader awareness—a mind open and perceptive—and there was space between problem-solving for reflection. It was perfect! I couldn't have picked a better situation for gaining wisdom.

What a difference it made to see my life from this point of

view! Once I could accept the limits of my life, then I could accept the gift within these limits.

Everyone has limits. Princess Di cannot have a temper tantrum, or go skinny dipping, or do mud wrestling and at least a few other things. The Pope cannot spend a night with the guys at the local tavern or enjoy playing raucously in a rock band. The President of the United States cannot say what he really thinks, nor can he walk alone under the moonlight or motorcycle across the country. Fashion models cannot enjoy eating, nor is it probable they can be presidents of colleges. And all famous people must watch their every public step, must put on smiles when they walk out of their houses no matter how they feel, must swallow their belches, must be what the public wants them to be. No person is without limits, free and able to do everything.

Besides the limits of our bodies, culture, and family leanings, time and space are themselves parameters of the game of life. There isn't time in one lifetime to do everything, and it isn't possible to be everywhere—hour by hour, we can only be "somewhere." But within our situations, something new and valuable is emerging. By standing joyfully inside our limits, we find that our eternal souls are able to expand.

The opportunities of each life are unique gifts to us alone. We prove ourselves adults and we reach a productive peace when we accept our opportunities, our challenges, and our gifts. In the language of another culture that took pride in living fully: "A warrior takes his lot, whatever it may be, and accepts it in ultimate humbleness. He accepts in humbleness what he is, not as grounds for regret but as a living challenge."[8]

We are born clay.

After some time
Pain begins to form us as a bowl.
The bowl will be
   the holder of our gifts.

We ourselves will fill the bowl
by accepting our gifts.

Pain creates the bowl.
Each bowl defines some limits,
   some closed doors.
The clay becomes shaped to hold
   a particular gift.

Usually
the bowl is small in the beginning;
though sometimes it's a right-away large bowl.
Sometimes it's small
and later grows larger,
And then later
perhaps larger still.

Pain creates the bowl
but Pain also holds the gift.
To receive the gift
we must stand up,
face Pain calmly and eye-to-eye,
and open our hands.
I say,

"I want my gift."
I say to you, Pain,
you who created my large bowl,
give me my large gift.

Thank you for the bowl that holds my gift,
the bowl that enables me to receive.
Thank you for the bowl with my limits,
my limits that define my special gift.

I say,
Thank you for my large gift.

III

Trying

13

Wishing for Magic

In the end, one must be one's own doctor. The will to wholeness and to health must come from within us.
—ELIZABETH WATSON

JUST AS SOME OF US WILL CHOOSE TO DIE FIGHTING rather than cooperate with the force of The Other whom we confront in pain, so some of us will also die rather than give up our little pleasures and habits. We are free to do this. The price for this choice, however, is pain.

In a society where comfort and pleasure are among the highest values, we can feel overwhelmed when we realize how much effort and discomfort we must experience to be free of pain. Perhaps we failed to respond to little pains, we ignored the warnings; as a result, the situation is now extreme. To make matters worse, we are unaccustomed to effort and discomfort. Now we find out what we are made of. We must remember that excuses rob us of power. In a society that doesn't encourage taking responsibility for ourselves—we pay experts to solve all our problems—pain asks us to take our lives in our hands and do all we can to save ourselves.

There *is* a magician: Grace. The Divine Presence loves and treasures and upholds us. We are guided and supported. But we must love ourselves as much as Life loves us. Only *we* can make the choices that will make our lives better. Wishing and choosing are not the same. Stephen Levine said the blunt truth of it: "Letting go of our suffering is the hardest work we will ever do."[1]

I like my pain.

Well, living with pain is easier than changing.
Changing is painful, too—
pain and pain, either direction.
I don't want to give up
   my little pleasures
   and familiar ways.
I'll die before I give them up!

I love the limitations of my pain.
They are excuses to do
   what I really want to do,
and excuses to not do
things I say I want to do,
or am told I should want to do
but don't really want to do.
Pain gives me an excuse.

Actually, I don't like my pain.
I wish it would go away like magic.
But if there's no magic,
I'd rather live with my pain
than change myself.

14

Trying Hard

Don't push the river—it flows by itself.
                                        —FRITZ PERLS

TOWARD WHAT DO WE DIRECT OUR EFFORT WHEN THE signs say that change wants to come?

Some of us are fighters and strugglers by nature; we'll do anything we can think of to conquer this problem. But there is such a thing as trying too hard and stumbling over our own feet. When the new is coming, it has its own force. The baby in the womb wants to be born; it's *determined* to be born, it will kill to be born. And the womb, too, wants to be rid of this pressure. Nature is with us. We don't need to fight, we just need to be sure we're directing our efforts with the flow of what's happening naturally.

Life is not as hard as we think. Nor is it easy: change *does* require effort. The mistake we often make—one that doubles the effort required—is to aim our effort in the wrong direction. We needn't force ourselves to change. We must aim toward relaxing the part of us that resists while focusing on the part

62

of us that wants to be born. There is no call for battle here, no need to kill something that's part of us. Trying to convince ourselves to kill a part of ourselves: this is a battle that our hearts can't fully embrace.

Remembering that we are born surrounded and upheld by Love, we direct our attention not toward a battlefield of good versus evil but toward a flow of energy called "growth," from the good to the better, from limitation to increase. We are part of the urge of the whole world toward an increase in beauty, power, wholeness, poise, fruitfulness, health, joy.

The safest path is one we don't have to walk alone. The path of communion with the loving Source of our lives may be rugged, but if we walk with the Source of all the power in the universe, in the end we cannot fail.

There are two streams in life. One is the stream of least resistance, the other is the Graced stream. The first is weighted with the power of our culture, our surroundings, our habits, and the conscience of our minds as it has been formed over the years. This is not necessarily the stream of health.

The other, the stream of Grace, is both hard and easy. We may for years have resisted our growth. Our shell of resistance to our growth is thick with habit, patterns, familiarity, comfort. Great effort is often needed to break free from these patterns. But this effort is different from doing battle; it requires simply that we gently hold our attention on the new that is trying to happen. As we focus on the new, our effort is very much like relaxing. To aim our effort toward relaxing the old and welcoming the new—this we can do successfully because it is an act of *loving ourselves,* not killing ourselves. It's more like sailing a boat: not pushing forward by brute force, but watching and moving with the wind, making use of the power that's blowing.

After an accident, Dr. Oliver Sacks found himself a helpless patient. His life's work had been conquering pain and illness, but now he learned that neither his usual assertiveness, nor his knowledge, nor his determination to get well—none of these could bring about his healing.

> . . . I had to relinquish all the powers I normally command. . . . above all, a sense of activity. I had to allow— and this seemed horrible—the sense and feeling of passivity. I found this humiliating at first, a mortification of myself. And then mysteriously, I began to change—to allow, to welcome, this abdication of activity. . . . The watchword at this time was "Be patient—endure ". . . . Wait, be still. . . . Do nothing, don't think! How difficult, how paradoxical, a lesson to learn![2]

May we do our doing wisely, not with brute force but with awareness. Sometimes it's better to do nothing than to do the wrong thing. And sometimes effort is not needed at all; Grace is ready and willing to carry us in a new direction. May we know when it's appropriate to "give up" and be held and carried by Love.

I grit my teeth and push forward.
I will not be conquered!
Or if I must fall
I'll fall heroic.
Effort—groan, grunt,
Pow!
Bang!
I'll make this change occur.
I'll try every path,
   take every treatment.
I know it all depends on me.
I am not a dreamer,
I'm the doer.
And I will do
and do and do and do and do. . . .

15

When Change Takes Time

Poppy petals fall softly,
quietly, calmly
when they are ready.

—ETSUJIN

CHANGE AND HEALING BRIDGE THE WORLDS OF ETER-
nity and time. We can invite them into our world of time and
matter. But they also belong to that large, uncontrollable world
of The Other, The Ruthless Force: we cannot command them
to come.

When pain lingers on like an unwanted guest who won't
leave, perhaps its business isn't finished. Pain may still be waiting for a chance to say something that's difficult to say. It's as
if you've talked about the weather, the economy, the news, all
the other relatives and neighbors, and what's wrong with the
rest of the world, but perhaps there's still some meat-and-
potatoes/close-to-home subject on which you haven't heard
the news.

Pain has more truth to tell us, and hard as it may be, that

truth is our only hope for freedom. Go back and listen some more. Without judging anything as good or bad, with no subjects protected from the truth, let us ask again with open hands what more gifts our pain wants to give us. Deeper and deeper levels of healing: gifts, gifts, and more gifts. When we've uncovered one, we're able to see the next.

Or perhaps we are caught halfway between the world of wishing and the world of really wanting. Does the thumbscrew have to turn tighter to convince us to change our path and really get a move on toward our healing? Where are we divided inside, trying to walk both north and south at the same time? Which part of our complex self is not yet convinced and happy about changing?

Must change and healing happen slowly? Yes and no. Human history is full of stories of moments of enlightenment and moments of physical healing. Even surgery, when successful in its goal, is instantaneous healing. The cripple who finally stands and walks has always been among us. Reconciliation between separated people, though not recorded as often as the separations, has happened a billion times.

Normally, our bodies change slowly, but they do change: the cells in our bodies are constantly dying and being replaced by new cells. According to Dr. Deepak Chopra,

> Ninety-eight percent of the atoms in your body were not there a year ago. . . . you acquire a new skeleton every three months. The skin is new every month. You have a new stomach lining every four days, . . . a new liver every six weeks."[3]

Our spirits are the motors that turn the direction of our bodies and also of the well-worn paths of our emotions and habits.

When the turn is happening imperceptibly, we must, with patience and persistance, keep our spirits in the positive direction. To turn back would be to lose the changes that are barely visible but building surely. A dear friend who lives beside the ocean described how she carefully watched the tide, trying to discern the exact moment when the water changed directions. She said it wasn't perceptible. The incoming tide became the outgoing tide at a moment so tiny the human eye could never see it. Beyond what the eye could see, the energy to change direction built gradually until, in one smallest movement, the whole direction changed. We never know how near we may be to that moment when the change we've been trying to make will begin to happen naturally.

Remembering that we are loved and we are not working alone toward our healing, this is an important time to ask for help from the Source of our Lives. We know that Love often brings surprises, Love can think and do things that we cannot imagine.

There's one change we can make that will significantly speed our healing: we can work at acting with confidence in our deepest intuitions, thus freeing the power of Grace to help us quickly and constantly.

At first this may feel like a leap into the dark; we haven't been taught that life is safe and that healing is always naturally trying to occur. We've been taught, rather, that rational thinking and our own control are the only safe bases for action. To act trusting in communion with a larger loving Power takes practice.

To be patient and non-judgemental toward ourselves will get us further on our path of progress. Decisions are not "right" and "wrong." We can try ideas, knowing that we are upheld and that nothing is a failure because we always learn and grow from whatever happens; learning and growing are our goals in being alive.

My pain is slow and reluctant to change direction.
My thoughts move quickly,
but my body and my emotions lag behind.
I don't want to feel what I feel.
My thoughts have improved;
my pain should be gone.

My feelings are awkward, disobedient;
they know a well-worn path.
My mind is light like the wind.
But my lifetime is gathered here—
a very large ship.
The heavy ship is nudged again and again by pain
and ever so slowly
changes direction.

To try an idea is to dabble one's toe in the water.
I have not yet *realized* the idea.
With each ache, I become more committed.
Pain, my lover/torturer, is convincing me.
My tears are like a river wearing away a rock.
   Each time I cry,
      some of "old ways" gets washed away.
   Yes, there is room for still another gift.

Or perhaps my pain has still more to say.
More words must come out.
My pain wants to say the whole truth;
it has so many things to say!
My words are balm on hurting wounds:

69

I hear my own words of truth;
My pain feels respected and can be still again.

The heavy ship bounces,
   then turns
      ever so slightly.
There is no other way to move this ship.
Time, time, time,
ache, pain, ache,
My heart is opening to a new way.

16

Progress

The crucial step cannot be taken until people are ready to choose the less which can be realized in place of the more which had remained a dream.

—L.L. WHYTE

MY SISTER-IN-LAW IS A PHYSICAL THERAPIST. ONE GREAT obstacle she encounters in patients with whom she works is imagination that is not balanced by realism. While dreaming about doing large things, people sometimes refuse to take the little steps. Imagination, in fact, is an important part of healing. We cannot do anything new if we can't imagine ourselves doing it. But imagination can be too strong for our own good; it can leap too far ahead of our actions. It should always stay connected to reality, like a shadow that falls just ahead of us as we walk.

When imagination runs too far in front, our focus is distracted away from the next step. And so we may never arrive at imagination's goal. Step by step is the only way to get to the dream.

71

Besides imagination, judgement can also be an enemy to healing. Good judgement is a servant who guides our doing. But often we let it become a tyrant who cares only about collecting a treasury of medals.

Life is an ongoing action. We must enjoy the "doing" of our life—each step, each moment, each challenge. Until we're dead, it's too soon to be counting our medals or judging our whole story. If our goal is just the end product, then each day, each step, is a dead experience. We must enjoy each step.

"Shoulds" are a particularly heavy judgement we lay on ourselves. Thinking that we "should" be able to do this or that hinders us from being happy in our small but real step-by-step progress.

Judgement too often compares. We may feel disheartened when we compare ourselves with others, or even with ourselves as we used to be. Runners on the outside of a circular track must not compare themselves with runners on the inside. All must simply run their very best from their own individual starting positions. Winning the race does not depend on the way things look to the eyes of the watchers. "Winning" depends simply on the amount of effort the runners are willing to exert to finish step-by-step to their own individual finish lines. In the end, we may have to pin the medal on our own chests, since no one else may know just how much effort it took for us to do something.

But the fact is, we *do* know. Let's not buy into "generic judgement." When we've taken one step that was very difficult, we can celebrate, congratulate ourselves, enjoy the sense of accomplishment. We can treat ourselves as kindly as we would treat a friend struggling with this problem.

When we live in our heads, in our imaginations, we turn our backs on our own selves. By accepting ourselves with love and mercy in the real present, we give ourselves a chance to have a real life.

Only we can do this. Only we can choose to really live or to pretend to live.

I made it!
  I conquered pain by an inch today!
One gigantic, ecstatic inch.

One of my eyes sees far ahead
  and imagines beating pain by miles:
playing tennis
  leaping on the beach
  climbing mountains.
I must put a patch over that eye;
it makes me so excited I can't take one step!

Perhaps someday I *will* beat pain by miles—
  or maybe I won't.

My only chance
  is to start with an inch
and enjoy the satisfaction
  of making it two inches.

I'll be glad to stretch myself another inch.
I'll be proud to make it from here to there.
If I focus close up,
  the *way* itself
  will be *full of joy*.

IV

Where We Are Free in Pain

17

Choices and Valuing

The importance of each minute decision by the most minor actor with the smallest bit part will influence all of the other actions both present, past, and future.
—WILLIAM JAMES

WHEN I WAS REALLY LOW AT ONE POINT IN MY LIFE, I made a collage from pictures found in magazines. The collage turned out to be a picture of the earth, and a large footprint in the sand, and the words "I was here. Does anybody remember me?"

Something in me was crying for an outlet, a voice. There is a creative urge in all of us; deep inside we know we have the power to make a difference somewhere to someone in perhaps some particular way. Until we find satisfying creative work we feel only half here.

But besides our unique callings, we are creating our world at every moment, creating our own experience, increasing or decreasing our own pain, affecting our relatives and friends and neighbors, our country, and our whole world. We throw a plastic bottle in the woods, and now there's a place where no plant will grow for a hundred years. In anger we call a child stupid, and the little trusting brain registers that like a fact: for years that brain remembers that it's "stupid." We cannot smile or frown without affecting those around us. If we choose to smoke this cigarette or not smoke this cigarette, to eat salad or pie, we take another step on a path toward a particular future.

We may choose to do something new and risky or not to try it, and so we either create new opportunities for ourselves or find ourselves in the same old place. We can choose to spend our time earning more money, or enjoying the company of people, or taking a course, or watching television, or helping someone in need, or doing something physical, or being alone. Each choice is okay, but each is a path leading away from goals that we could reach on other paths. We are creating our lives. The more we put energy into anything the more we increase the future chance of more of this happening.

Our example affects everyone we touch. We choose to tell a lie, and everyone who knows this feels more inclined to lie. We vote or we don't vote, and so our government becomes ours or is free of our influence, and our neighbors are more inclined or less inclined to vote. We choose to follow a tradition or stand against it, and so the tradition is strengthened or weakened, and others notice our example and feel pulled.

Someone hurts us, and we choose to make a big deal of it or a small deal of it: our own pain increases or decreases by our choice. Someone hurts us, and we choose to speak up or remain silent: if we remain silent the person never knows he or she hurt us and never changes, and may go on to hurt someone else, and we may get an ulcer and feel smaller.

We are part of group decisions—to go to war or not to go to war, decisions to join the trend and buy and sell people as slaves, to cooperate and pay taxes to England or not to, to

78

accept pornography as "normal" or not to, to become involved with what's happening in Germany, Pakistan, China, Sudan, or Guatemala, or to decide to stay out of those people's lives.

If we are the ones affected by a group decision—we are the one who lost his legs in Viet Nam, was raped by someone stimulated by pornography—it is important to the group that we speak up and give feedback: "Hey! This idea hurts! This idea is not healthy for living, growing things. . . ." We may be tempted to think that the group won't listen. But if it's not said, it can't be heard. We create the world when we remain silent about our pain. We give a green light to hurtful actions, patterns, laws, ideas. Or, if we speak up, we move the world in an ever-so-slight change of direction. The earth is big, groups of people are big, but with enough nudges anything can move.

The earth will never forget that we were here. We create ourselves, other people, and the earth itself by our choices. We do this by whatever we choose to value. Things that are valued increase; things that are not valued decrease. How do we know what to value? By pleasure and pain. Is this pleasing or displeasing to us? We assign the value to what we are given and what we experience.

Scientists are not in agreement on whether our galaxy is expanding or contracting. That's because we haven't made up our minds yet on whether we want to expand it or contract it. We are creators: each choice for safety contracts all; each act of courage expands the universe.

We create the universe
  by what we value.
We say: "Let there be . . .
        Let there not be. . . ."
We throw our energy into this flow or that.
We throw our energy against
  the flow that displeases us.
We create the world
by our choices.

Pain is our guide as we create the universe.
We experiment.
And we are part of experiments.
Our feedback is important:
We cry out to Grace, "This hurts!
Forget this idea!"

We create ourselves by choices we make.
We increase or decrease our own experiences.
In one moment, something crosses our path.
We can re-member that one moment
  over and over and over,
    multiplying the size of the experience,
      multiplying its power,
Or we can leave its power behind,
  isolated to that moment.
Valuing this,
believing in that,
seeking more . . . ,
hanging onto . . . ,

80

trying to be rid of . . . ,
We take what we are given
and consume it for its passing value
or increase it by our added attention.

We dialogue with the given.
Homesteaders or Gypsies,
we survey what we find,
decide to cling to it, identify with it—
"this is me, this is home"—
or we take what there is of joy and value
and move on lightly to the new.
We carry what baggage we choose to carry.

I've chosen the setting for today's experience.
I am choosing the setting for tomorrow.
I create the world in which experience comes to me.
I value this and not that.
The universe expands (or contracts) by my choices.

18

Pain Is a Measuring Cup

*By going along with feelings you unify your emotional,
mental and bodily state. When you try to fight or deny
them, you divorce yourself from the reality of your being.
[Accepting them] at least roots you firmly in the integrity
of your present experience and allows its innate motion and
natural creativity to thrust toward a therapeutic solution.*
—SETH

JUST AS PAIN IS A MIRROR IN WHICH WE SEE INVISIBLE
truths about ourselves, so pain is a measuring cup in which
we can see truths about our relationships.

When my husband died unexpectedly, I felt as if my heart
had been ripped open by a dagger and my chest was an open
wound. I was in such shock and grief I couldn't eat or sleep.

But after some time I became aware of a little corner inside
me that was curious: how much *did* I really love this man?
We had our differences, as every married couple does. Many
times I'd felt frustrated and angry with him. Were we really
as happy as I'm now thinking we were?

Instinctively, I let myself feel what I honestly felt. There was no other way to know what size of gift this person had been.

As I began to make decisions after his death, I began to know. I found that I was unable to allow an autopsy or donate his organs: no matter what my head said, my feelings dictated that this body was sacred. And then I found myself holding his warm body in my arms for four hours. The hospital was anxious to put this "thing" in cold storage, but for me it was still the connecting link to a treasured presence that was quickly leaving me.

As time went on, my curious corner watched with surprise as months, years came and went, and tears would still come unexpectedly. Always different, but still the sense of something treasured that was missing.

It was actually harder to allow myself to start laughing again. But honest laughter was important, too. Both the tears and the laughter together mark the boundaries of "exactly what this person meant to me."

Tom died at 1:30 A.M. on Labor Day weekend. The next day the school year would begin; our two teenage children decided not to miss the beginning of classes. I let them follow their own intuitions. I respected their right to absorb this event in their own time and manner.

Other people told them what they could expect to feel: "You have to cry to be healthy." I told them not to let anyone tell them what to feel. They knew they were free to cry. And what he meant to me as a husband could be different from what he meant to each of them—a boy and a girl—as a father. There is an integrity in honesty that enables the surest healing of whatever wants healing.

Did we have a happy marriage? With death, the tendency is to remember only good and happy moments, feeling ashamed of any angry memories. With divorce and break-ups one remembers only bad and unhappy moments, not knowing what to do with the good memories. But lest any truth get lost, it seems valuable to allow contradictory feelings to co-exist and sort themselves out. Somewhere in the strange mess there is "truth." We will learn much more if we don't judge what we're feeling as good or bad, right or wrong, but just watch what honestly comes and goes. After the dust settles, we can see what's there and decide what to do with it if we feel like doing something.

Pain is a measuring cup
through which we see value.
When something is taken away,
do we miss it a little or a lot?
Truly or pretend?
How much did it weigh—
   are we heavier without it or lighter?
How big was it—
   how big is the space that's left when it's gone?
How long does it take to fill the space up again?
How much of myself is missing
   when this part of my life
     is torn out of me?
How many moons does it take
to get back in balance?
How much strength does it take
   to put one foot in front of the other
     and continue walking?
Is my pain really there?
Or is it an illusion of invisible oughts and wants?
     Is it solid, or is it air?

19

Re-membering the Sweet

*"To me, you are still nothing more than a little boy who
is just like a hundred thousand other little boys. . . .To you,
I am nothing more than a fox like a hundred thousand
other foxes. But if you tame me, then we shall need each
other. To me, you will be unique in all the world . . . it
will be as if the sun came to shine in my life. . . . look: you
see the grain-fields down yonder? I do not eat bread. Wheat
is of no use to me. The wheat fields have nothing to say to
me. And that is sad. But you have hair that is the color
of gold. Think how wonderful that will be when you have
tamed me! The grain, which is also golden, will bring me
back the thought of you. And I shall love to listen to the
wind in the wheat. . . ."*

*So the Little Prince tamed the fox. And when the hour
of his departure drew near—*

"Ah," said the fox, "I shall cry."

*"It is your own fault," said the little prince. "I never
wished you any sort of harm; but you wanted me to tame
you . . . it has done you no good at all!"*

*"It has done me good," said the fox, "because of the color
of the wheat fields."*

—ANTOINE DE SAINT EXUPERY

86

ONE OF MY REACTIONS AFTER TOM'S DEATH WAS TO SCOUR the house for photographs of him and to put aside countless items that carried precious memories. I put a good bit of time into this, but it felt therapeutic. Each time I found a new picture I'd cry because the photo would bring back the sense of his presence. But gradually each photo receded once again into "just a photo"; thus little by little I accustomed myself to the distance between us.

I actually had the sense that in some way Tom was participating in this: that "being dead" required adjustment on his part, too, and that we were both properly and temporarily focused now on memories. What had this life of his been about? For him it would be a self-evaluation and a reaping of the harvest of his doing; for me it was a summarizing of the gift that he had been to me.

Even more, for me it was a way of trying to stay in touch with him. And I knew with my rational mind that somewhere down the road this activity would have to end. One cannot look backward forever, and there was no way for us to go forward together now; our paths were parting. I knew that some day in the future I would have to make the terrible choice to stop re-membering him. I dreaded this; I couldn't imagine not thinking about him, because that would seem the end of his being in my life.

But I've come to recognize that Tom is always in my life, whether I think about him or not. All of life has a different quality after someone has truly loved us. The world we walk in is *always* richer and more beautiful, whether that person is with us still or not. As the Fox told the Little Prince, the wheat fields would always be more beautiful because of him. The pain we feel over losing the presence of a person is a reminder of the value of what we've been given.

But just as there had been an importance to our being together, my mind knew there was also some importance to our separation. Eventually I would have to become the separated person Life was asking me to be.

Physical separation can happen quickly, but psychological separation takes time. There's no need to rush. Good memories continue to give blessings. But a happy story that's ended is a double-edged blessing: the painful side is valuable because it pushes us away from what is trying to end. This pain is like a guide, like an angel who gently but firmly steers us toward a new path. We cannot stand to feel grief forever, and so at some point we let go of looking backward and let the pain be lifted off our shoulders. We are forced eventually to turn toward life, to open to new joy, to go on growing, to face our new challenges and opportunities.

Pain is often the only window
through which the treasured (or awful) past
can be kept in the present.
I love my pain
because it is the blessed medium
through which I see you and touch you
when you are far away.
It is the sacred link that keeps us together
when time and space keep us apart.

O pain that doubles my joy!
Now you, O dear one, are gone,
and no more adventures will be added to our story.
So I remember.
I live again every wonderful moment.
If I put away these happy memories
and look at them no more
I'll be free of pain.
But oh, such wonderful times we had!
I want to relish them again.
I want to turn them over in my hand,
every little treasure you gave me.
Each time I look at them I know how rich I am.
And because I want to enjoy them again
I accept the pain of remembering.
My pain is an act of treasuring.
My pain is my reward.
I worked hard to build a precious thing,

and it was taken from me.
I worked and sacrificed for the best,
and the best came to me.
Now my loss is great!
I loved with all my heart,
not half a heart,
and now my whole heart is broken!

I love my pain:
It is the shadow always with me
of my great blessing.

20

When Others Value Me

"Go and look again at the roses. You will understand now that yours is unique in all the world. . . ."

The little prince went away, to look again at the roses. . . . And the roses were very much embarassed. . . . "An ordinary passerby would think that my rose looked just like you—the rose that belongs to me. But in herself alone she is more important than all the hundreds of you other roses: because it is she that I have watered; because it is she that I have put under the glass globe; because it is she that I have sheltered behind the screen; because it is for her that I have killed the caterpillars (except the two or three that we saved to become butterflies); because it is she that I have listened to, when she grumbled, or boasted, or even sometimes when she said nothing. Because she is my rose."

[Said the fox], . . ." It is the time you have wasted for your rose that makes your rose so important. . . . You become responsible, forever, for what you have tamed. You are responsible for your rose. . . ."

—Antoine de Saint Exupery

EARLY IN OUR MARRIAGE MY HUSBAND WAS IN THE HOS-pital recovering from heart surgery when a terrible train crash occurred. Two passenger trains hit head on. Many of the injured were brought to the hospital where Tom was. After a few days, he took his intravenous contraption and shuffled down the hall to visit.

He found one young woman who had been hanging upside down for six hours before they could cut her out. Her jaw was broken, teeth smashed, legs broken, hips broken, and so on. When her mother had walked into the room to identify her she had turned to leave because she didn't recognize her daughter. Sue had so many operations to face that the surgeons hardly knew where to begin.

And—her fiance had been hanging dead beside her.

Sue said to Tom as they talked, "If only he had lived. I would have a reason to go through all this recovery!"

Tom thought for a minute. He had faced death now, along with the wonder of what might be the meaning of his life if he were to die so young. He had asked himself what he had given to the world, and he had answered it.

So he said to her, "When two people marry, the basic gift that they give to each other is an affirmation: 'This is what I think you're worth—I will give my whole life to helping you. You are worth all that I have to give.' When your fiance promised to marry you, didn't he give you that affirmation then? Didn't he tell you how much you're worth? Then accept his gift, and take care of your self, who is worth so much."

Sometimes the Love that upholds all life comes to us directly, and sometimes it comes through others: parent, spouse, teacher, neighbor, friend, fireman, counselor, nurse. Particularly when choices must be made: we should not forget or belittle the actions that lean in our favor and cost another. Every act of love that anyone's ever done for us told us that we are valuable.

If right now we find ourselves alone, we can remember all the love that others have given us over the years. It may be true that some people *didn't* love us, or didn't love us in a way that felt healthy. We can decide either to remember those who valued us or to focus on those who didn't, to remember all the acts of love or the failures in love. If we remember these moments when we were valued we increase the influence of all the good that's come into our lives.

Your choices tell me what you think I'm worth.
I remember things you sacrificed for me
because you valued me.
I said I needed something—
you dropped what you were doing to help me.
You were tired,
but you helped me
with warmth and gentleness.
Your scarce and precious time
you gave to me
when you could have used it for yourself.
I wanted to go here
and you wanted to go there,
and you chose me over you.
You didn't count the cost to you.
You paid the price of being with me in life
and proclaimed my value.
No one can make me feel like nothing now.
I will value your sacrifice
by taking care of myself.
You said I was loveable,
I was worth loving,
and so I will value and love myself.

21

I Value Myself

I shelter myself; in me is the house,
I guard myself and in me is the guard.
Beloved that I have become, on me rests
the lovely image of creation, crying itself out.
                    —RAINER MARIA RILKE

SOMETIMES WE DIG OURSELVES DEEPER INTO LONELI-
ness by looking only outside ourselves for love. We grab without heed at empty promises; we hope for love where there is
no sound basis for hope. We try to "make" others love us. But
our desperate acts are often repulsive and make others move
away from us.

We may be angry because we've not received from others
the love that we believe should have been given us. Negligent
or abusive or non-existent parents, cruel teachers, the spouse
that promised and then walked away, the lover that walked
on by—these people by their choices have said, "I do not value
you."

And so, because of others' actions—can we never feel our

95

value? We often say to ourselves, "I have low self-esteem because *X* didn't love me."

When others fail to value us, we have the opportunity to think for ourselves. We can either buy into others' judgements or make our own judgement. Because we know we are valuable, it is healthy to feel anger at others' neglect.

But excuses rob us of power. In all the universe, who is most responsible for me?

I am. It may be difficult to love ourselves without the affirmations that others take for granted. But it is not impossible.

The seeming isolation of individual experience is not because we are islands in the universe: we are part of each other and part of a whole. But "I" am the awareness that coordinates this unique set of experiences. I am responsible to care for them and bring fruit from them, to treasure and enjoy this once-in-the-universe life-force called "me." It is my responsibility, and I *can* do it.

We have the right to love ourselves.

We have the responsibility to love ourselves.

We may have to break with some traditional ideas about the dangers of loving ourselves too much. Most of us have to work in the opposite direction and try to achieve a normal, healthy self-love. How can we love anyone else until we're also convinced of our own worth? First things must come first. Whitney Houston affirmed this responsibility in a popular song:

I found the greatest love of all
inside of me. . . .
learning to love yourself
is the greatest love of all.[1]

I feel pain
because no one has valued me.
No one.
There's a hole in me
that longs and reaches out:
"Oh value me, oh value me.
Oh give me some of your time, attention,
sacrifice just a little for me."
I long to hear someone tell me
what I already think:
I have value!
Yes, my pain tells me that I know it already.
The silence of the world
forces me to say it for myself:
I am a treasure.
Is everyone waiting for me to say it first?
My pain is confusion—
I thought someone else should say it first.
But the pressure of pain pushes me forward;
finally, I must be the first to say the truth:
"I am a *treasure!*"

22

Sacrifice and Bitterness

Hate does not affect the object being hated, but tears apart the vessel carrying it.

—TOM MCDONALD, QUOTING AN
UNREMEMBERED SOURCE

A FOG OF RELATED PAINS ROSE UP BEFORE ME ON A MARSH of heavy experiences. The pains asked me to find clarity and meaning among them. I could discern only a couple of words in the mist: sacrifice, bitterness.

I know a little of these. Most of us do. But how to understand them, how to stand under them and lift up their heaviness? How to redeem them for their gifts?

I decided to strike out into the world like a wandering reporter, to see whether the world itself understood these better than I. "I'll ask anyone: everyone knows something about these."

So I went next door and inquired of Wes and Leah if they knew anything about sacrifice or bitterness. At eighty years, Wes is still enjoying life, friendly, kind, married to his warm and loving childhood sweetheart Leah after both were widowed. "Yes," they said, "we know a little about these subjects."

When Wes was eleven, his father, a painter, was paralyzed by the arsenic absorbed from paint fumes. Wes had five younger brothers and sisters. There was no choice: he must quit school and help his Mom support the family, living on a rented 320-acre farm. The boy sat down with his Mom to calculate what they were going to do. This eleven-year old went to the bank in their small town where the banker knew them and presented the family plan and the calculation of the amount the family needed to borrow. The banker asked Wes if he knew how to purchase the milk cows he wanted to buy, and Wes assured him he did. "Go pick them out and bring me the note," the banker said.

Besides five small children, Wes's mother raised from two to three thousand chickens. The chicken farm succeeded except for the loss from a Kansas tornado, when three hundred chickens lost their feathers and were plastered into a mesh fence! Funny now. At the end of five years Wes had built a herd of forty-five cattle and every year raised 4,000 bushels of wheat and 5,500 bushels of corn.

When Wes's father was paralyzed, he asked his Dad if he was going to have to quit school. Tears came to his Dad's eyes, so Wes never asked him again. The doctors said there was no hope for the man to recover, but his Dad turned his attention intently toward trying to move himself. He would grab the curtain and inch his hand painfully up the wall. After five years of determined effort, Wes's dad went back to work as a painter.

Wes had been a whiz in math all through elementary school and wanted to study engineering. He had an uncle who owned a store in a college town and had promised Wes a place to stay when the boy would go to college. But Wes was sixteen when his dad returned to work and felt too embarassed to return to school being so far behind his peers.

For five years Wes wandered around the country feeling

bitter. He covered thirty-nine states and worked in oil fields, wheat fields, orchards, coal mines, stores. He kept wandering, trying to find a way out of his bitterness. Finally he fell into a job with a gas company that required intelligence but not a degree. He studied at night and was able to do this work, finding it challenging and satisfying, and his bitterness began to leave him.

"I had lost something I felt I should have had," Wes explained to me. "It was nobody's fault; there was nobody in particular to feel bitter toward. My bitterness left once I found satisfying work. I just gave up judging it as wrong, so I let go of it. I was proud to be able to help my family, and the bond and understanding between my Mom and me became really strong.

"My father had a sister named Mary," Wes went on. "Her husband run off and left her when their kids were small. She ended up raising three families: her daughter died leaving two little boys, and then one of those boys was killed and left a couple more great-grandkids for her to raise. She was still raising kids when she was eighty years old. She was jolly. She was glad to do it. At eighty-eight she fell and broke both hips. The doctor said she'd never mend, but after a year she was right up walking again.

"But I have a sister, Faye," Wes continued. "Her husband and her son and her daughter-in-law all died within five years of each other. The son was her only child. That happened twenty-five years ago, but she's still bitter. Nobody can get along with her. But she was selfish to begin with; she just goes on being nasty and bitter."

Leah has her own story. When she was three months old, her mother died in a fire. Her father's sister and her mother's sister both wanted to adopt her, but her father wouldn't allow it; instead, he gave her to his own mother to raise. His mother was twice widowed already; she had had six children by her first marriage, only two of them reaching adulthood. By the

100

time she took baby Leah she was alone raising two young sons.

Leah's grandma was sad in spirit and very protective, always afraid that something bad would happen. Leah wasn't allowed to run and play like other children and had an unnaturally quiet childhood.

Leah's father never came to visit, except once when she was five. She remembers that a man came whom she guessed must be her father, but she had to inquire in private, since she didn't know what her father looked like.

For years Leah was bitter toward her father. But she knew the past would never get talked about or worked out; there was no going back. So she finally gave up on the bitterness: it was too heavy and self-destructive.

I talked with other members of Leah's family; they, too, had suffered deep hurts and injustices. As I talked with them, instead of seeing a family with lots of troubles I see the whole human race. I'm sure that if I continued asking, everyone in the world would have something truly sad to tell me, and they would not be soap-opera exaggerations but true experiences of injustice or deprivation. We all truly have justifiable reasons for bitterness.

"But are all these situations the same?" I ask myself. "Can we just point our finger at Wes's sister Faye for clinging to her bitterness and give a medal to Wes and Leah, who've let go of theirs? Is this all there is to say?"

I notice one difference between Wes's story and that of Faye: Wes's loss enabled good to come to others. He could see some value in his suffering. Similarly, his jolly Aunt Mary had the satisfaction of seeing the hardships she endured enable several children to reach adulthood. This I would call sacrifice. We give of ourselves so that good may come to others. In the end, it can actually give us joy to know that, although we suffered, our existence made a difference in the world.

When our giving is not done in freedom but is instead taken

101

from us, we are justified in our bitterness. But the value of our acts helps ease the pain of our loss. Faye could not find this value in her suffering; her loss did not seem to bring benefit to anyone.

But the same could be said of Leah's pain.

Bitterness is unfair by its nature. One may be totally justified in feeling bitter toward others or toward life; yet to continue in this feeling never corrects the wrong and hurts no one but one's own self.

Bitterness increases the size of the wrong done to us. Each time we re-member the wrong, we give it life again. We give our oppressor power over us many times stronger than the original wrong done so long ago.

In the end, it appears to me that bitterness is a small knife by which we slowly kill ourselves. In the ignorance of our egos we feel that we are loving ourselves, but we've actually become our own oppressors. Our hearts become hard and heavy from carrying bitterness. Our anger eats at us. We close ourselves off from new joy and love, allowing the resentment to keep the past in the place where the present should be.

Beth, Leah's granddaughter, had been married six years when her husband left her for another woman. Her brother, Ken, said to his sister—with love and with the simplicity of the young—"Your life is like a bathtub, and he's just pulled the plug. Your tub used to be full and warm and soapy and comfortable. Now it's empty and hard and cold. But *you* can put the plug back in! And God will fill up your tub again. Maybe even to overflowing! Other people will pull your plug; it will happen every now and then in life. Just learn to re-member to quickly put the plug right back in, and then accept what's coming in to fill it. . . ."

"Now I understand something more about sacrifice and bitterness," I think to myself. "But why am I unable to let go

102

of my own bitterness?" The source of my own bitterness seems objectively small, in comparison with the serious injustices done to others.

When I was in high school, I mustered the nerve one day to ask my father a wish that was deep in my heart. "When I go to college," I began shyly, "do you think I could go to the University of Michigan?" The big University of Michigan, the place of mystique in my mind, where learning is taken seriously, where I might dig deeply into learning as I longed to do.

My father thought for a short minute, and said a slow no. . . . "You'd just be a little fish in a big sea," he said. His sister had gone from a small town like ours to the big Michigan State and was terribly homesick the first year; he didn't want me to suffer as she had. In fact, she had adjusted and graduated happily from there. But my loving father did not want to see me endure what she had undergone in her freshman year.

So the river of my life had to find some other course. I floundered around. I entered a convent to be a nun and was very unhappy. I studied music and failed miserably. I left the convent, married, and raised children—the things that "women do." I loved my children, but I always had a tinge of bitterness inside, a feeling that my life had been taken from me and that what I was doing wasn't really me.

I did do many interesting things over the years, and I continued to study and learn. But thirty years later, I still hear this pain inside me whining, "But I didn't get to go to the University of Michigan."

My judgement says this is silly, but logic doesn't seem to cure the painful longing. Why can't I say with Leah, "there's no going back, no way to fix the hurts of the past, so I'll just let go of my bitterness"?

Why does my will have a direction of its own? My will *wants* my bitterness. Why?

"Because you could still do it," says that shy voice inside.

103

"The U. of M. is still there. And you aren't dead yet. If you can't let go of your bitterness, go back and do the darn thing!"

Well, what a thought! It seems that time has finally carried me on my convoluted path to where I'm free to try whatever I want! Now I could go back and fix the hurting hole in my past. As a realistic friend said to me, I can still go back to study, I just can't be a cheerleader. . . .

Tears come to my eyes as I open to the possibility of healing this old pain. My bitterness has kept my dream alive. All these years, the hard shell of my bitterness has protected the tender seed of my hope.

I say thanks to this strange movement that goes on inside us called "bitterness." It is an instinct that desires to protect us, to keep us looking for the healthy path.

But like a friendly-but-ferocious watchdog, wisdom must grab the reins when bitterness points toward possible danger. If the watchdog runs the show, even the dog's owner could be hurt.

There is a large and dynamic power plant
   that faces maybe East or maybe West.

Looking West it sees the sunset.
The beautiful sun—
     haunting,
     looking glorious
     as it moves away beyond our reach.
The power plant watches the sunset intensely,
longingly.
It's slipping away!
And it was so beautiful.

What-might-have-been.

Sadness. Tightness. Anger. Bitterness.
The power slows down.
It stagnates. Or it burns up inside.
"If only. . . ."
"I had to. . . ."
"I couldn't. . . ."
    And it was all so beautiful.
What-might-have-been looks golden,
What was taken from me looks gigantic.
Robbery! Life stole it away.
Blackmail. I was forced to do it.
On the outside, paint tightens and peels and drops.
Inside wheels tighten, output slows
as attention is riveted
on the beautiful disappearing sun.

105

Looking East, the power plant sees
the sun is rising.
Energy is expanding in the universe!
Energy ignites energy.
What-might-be-for-us
   is coming up!

A thrill
to have the opportunity
to share something,
that my existence in the world makes a difference,
that my riches can enrich you, too.
I rejoice that there is us:
in my giving I know I'm not alone.
Oh the joy of having something to give,
of being able to give,
that someone wants what I have to give!

Facing East,
the power plant feels ecstasy and excitement:
I and the sun and the world are one!
The sun is coming to me
   with a new day and new energy.
I open my arms
and in comes always-flowing life,
and out it goes.
And the world around me turns better
because of the giving of my joyful energy,
because I am here.

23

Big Little-pains

No one can make you feel inferior without your consent.
—ELEANOR ROOSEVELT

ONCE (OR TWICE) MY DAUGHTER WAS HAVING PROBLEMS in her love life. Someone asked her if she was unhappy.

"I'm unhappy," she said, "but I'm not unhappy that I'm unhappy." In other words, "I'm not worrying about my state—I'm O.K.—you needn't worry about me."

We needn't be gobbled up by our own emotional reaction. A little pain is not a threat; even a big pain is not a threat, unless we cannot trust the ebbs and flows of natural life. When our bodies have been attacked or wounded, they immediately begin to mend themselves. When emotional health feels attacked, our psyches will also begin to move toward emotional healing. It will happen automatically if we're patient and if we neither fear nor suppress what we're feeling.

When our physical bodies are under major attack we may look for the help of a medical doctor to assist our body's natural healing. Likewise, under great emotional trauma, we may want

107

to seek professional help in our emotional healing. But healing always begins by nature itself, and we can cooperate with this natural process.

One thing we can do is to not give our own weight to the real or imagined intention of another to hurt us. Things that are valued increase; things that are not valued decrease. If I give value to another's bad actions, I *give that person continued power over me*. Every time I remember the action, I re-member—give body again—to that same action. It's as if by my choice I make it happen again and again.

Nothing in life *has* to leave us with life-long scars. Effects remain only as long as we don't accept the gift—that is, rise to the stronger place where we are in command of our reaction. First we must embrace the whole event as it happened—the pain inflicted on us, our reaction, our inability to cope; then we can begin to change its effect in us. We can react now in our imagination with our current wisdom, saying and doing what we now feel to be appropriate, not with bitterness but with blessing. While loving the self who struggled in ignorance, we realize we have learned. Our pain has lifted us into a new place, and we needn't re-member this over and over any more.

"When your memory goes—then you can forget it," says a funny button in the store. Our memories are our own storehouses; we draw from them what we want. With just a bit of effort, we can focus our attention on happy memories instead of on sad memories.

Tears have an immensely important power in the natural healing of emotions. The quickest way to get on with life is to let the tears flow without judgement or restraint. Tears give us an immediate measurement of what exactly has happened to us and how big it is, and they free us from the tension that builds around a confusion; they enable us to see clearly.

A friend of mine reached a relationship with his tears that

seems workable in a public life where crying is sometimes not possible. He says sometimes he doesn't need to cry, he just needs to get in touch with his tears. There was a time when he was letting go and catching up and could cry freely.

"I had access to my tears then; I learned how to cry. Now I've forgotten and I can't, and that's O.K. Sometimes now my eyes get wet, and I just feel the tears inside my chest. It's almost as if I can't grow if I don't feel my tears, as if the tears are connected with the idea that I'm cut. If I don't know where I'm cut, I don't know where to grow." For Tom Forsythe, the fruit of feeling his pain instead of running from it has been the beautiful poetry he's able to write.

If we feel attacked we needn't pretend that we're not wounded. But we needn't keep opening our own wounds again, nor need we fear what has happened. Nor do we need to create an armor around us against further attacks, because we are all the mythological cats with nine lives. We can be wounded again and again and not be killed, and we can actually be richer each time we're wounded! As long as we stay aware of what we're experiencing and cooperate with the natural processes that will heal us, then every wound has the possibility to make us larger, stronger, warmer; every wound can be a step deeper into our humanness.

The size of my pain appears very small,
but to me it feels big.
Its length is short, its mass is tiny,
but it feels dense and weighty.
I feel attacked unaware—
as if a small knife stabbed me,
was drawn out again,
and the culprit ran off in the shadows.
I will recover;
I'm only thrown off balance.
But it hurts greatly.
This was not a scratch:
someone touched a very sensitive nerve,
a vulnerable place.
But I'm strong enough.
And I know the way of power for healing wounds:
the natural way—a few drops of tears
administered immediately,
and I'll be back in balance,
but more alert this time
to take care of myself.
I will make this pain my ally;
I will turn this wound into liquid gold
to increase my warmth and power.
I will turn it into a hill and climb it
until I stand bigger and stronger on top of it.

24

Work, Work, Work

*The serious person is the one who thinks the environment
is more important than one's self; the playful person thinks
that the self is more important than the environment.*
—Jean Paul Sartre

ONE YEAR AFTER WE WERE MARRIED IT WAS DISCOV-
ered that my husband had Hodgkin's Disease, cancer of the
lymph system. We spent the first several years of marriage
going through radiation, surgery, and chemotherapy.

We got to the other side of all that, but we were not un-
changed. One effect I saw in Tom was a determination to
enjoy every minute of his life. He seemed to have decided
subconsciously, "If most of my life is going to be work, and
perhaps my life may be short, I'm going to enjoy whatever
I'm doing." He also did his best at whatever he did and then
refused to worry about what he couldn't control.

What upset him most was working with people who worked
with deadly seriousness. If co-workers couldn't joke a little,
he lost his enthusiasm for the project. Once in awhile he got

111

himself in trouble by his lightness when he was working with the deadly serious or with those who thought themselves amazingly important. But mostly his lightness gave energy to long days of work. After his death, a friend and co-worker said of Tom, "He enjoyed every day as a gift."

As I look back at these years, I realize that I was one of those who worked with deadly seriousness. And I was raising children! How can one raise little children and not be playful? It takes grim determination to fight the natural joy of the situation! I suppose I was focusing more on the outcome of the work than on the doing. So years of "hard work" passed for me while Tom was "having fun" at the office! It's not the work, it's the point of view. . . .

We've lost ourselves when the object of our doing becomes more important than the subject who's doing it. Our workplaces are the gardens in which we may grow to maturity in our humanness, in which we can reach our enlightenment, our personal power, our holiness, wisdom—whatever our soul considers great. Each workplace offers opportunities and challenges for us to become bigger people.

I've heard people blame the bureaucracy around them for their inability to be themselves at work, but structures are built and maintained by living people who all have the same urges and needs inside them. If we find the courage to try to function as real human beings in our workplaces, we may find that others want to be their real human selves, too. Someone must be the leader and start the tide turning. If we begin being real and not shells or facades, we'll find followers one by one and build communities around ourselves that are the healthy places in which we want to work.

Sometimes our work can feel like an awful burden. Then it isn't invigorating us but instead is draining us. We assume it's the job, the situation, the people with whom we work, the "bureaucracy" that controls us, the culture we live in, and so on. But the whole situation could feel different if we changed ourselves, and that is within our control to do. A friend of mine, Sister Barbara Blake, wrote a story for this situation.

A middle-aged warrior queen had recently fallen on hard times. In the past few years her kingdom had begun to crumble: crops were dying, the land was overrun with locusts, famine was near, neighboring armies were attacking, and her once-loyal troops were deserting. To the once-confident queen, all seemed hopeless. Her nights were sleepless, her energy low, and her manner agitated.

She decided to seek guidance at a holy place far distant from her kingdom. She left her royal robes behind and, with only a small knapsack, set out on her arduous journey on foot.

After months of lonely travel, she eventually reached the foothills of the sacred mountains and began her climb toward the holy peak. For days she pulled and dragged herself over gnarled roots and jagged rocks until she found the summit. There she encountered the wise old woman she had travelled so far to see.

The exhausted queen explained to the wise woman how she had worked and fought and struggled to keep her kingdom together. She had consulted with all the wise people of her realm, she was awake nights thinking and worrying, but nothing seemed to help. She pleaded with the wise woman to tell her what to do to save her kingdom.

The old woman silently lit an oil lamp, sprinkled sage in a circle around the queen, and intoned a low chant. Instantly the skies darkened, the winds blew fiercely, the clouds crackled with lightning. At that moment a small golden box appeared at the feet of the amazed queen. Ea-

113

gerly she opened the box to find inside a small note folded in half. Trembling, she unfolded the mysterious message. Two words were written in bold print:

LIGHTEN UP![2]

Work, work, work.
I feel sorry for myself.
My life is hard.
I'm tired.
And sad.
My pain is pity for poor me.
I used to have time for fun, for enjoying life.
Now work consumes my days.
How can I go on without joy and fun?

My guide, pain, says to me,
    "my challenge to you is this:
      make your work your fun!
Your mistake is to separate work and joy.
Enjoy the people around you.
Joke with them.
Learn to love them, be loyal to them as friends.
Treat them as you would like to be treated.
Learn to relax while working.
A happy attitude and relaxed body
will re-energize themselves.
Find a positive attitude toward the work you do;
feel satisfaction from your contribution and accomplish-
ment.
If you can't do this,
find the work about which you *can* feel positive.
And find the workplace where you can enjoy the people
around you.

Fun is whatever you decide is fun.
Either change your attitude
or change your situation.

(or continue in your pain. . . .)"

25

Little Heartbreak

When we begin to take our failures non-seriously, it means we are ceasing to be afraid of them. It is of immense importance to learn to laugh at ourselves.
—KATHERINE MANSFIELD

AT TIMES WE ALL GROPE AROUND WONDERING "AM I being true to myself?" "Who *is* my real self?" I find inside me two opposites that for years have confused my attempts to be clear about who I am. I've come to call these opposite parts of myself my Commonness and my Uniqueness. We all have both; perhaps we're each more comfortable with one than the other. But as we grow, we need to alternately embrace each of these parts because they complement each other and keep us balanced.

Our uniqueness can be frightening, because it seems to separate us from others. When we feel how we're different from everyone around us we can feel tempted to loneliness, or the rest of the world may seem illogical and threatening because we feel so different. But if we live only in our commonness, if we stay part of the crowd too much, we may feel unappreciated for our true selves; we can feel stifled, hidden, not really known or truly loved.

In moments of embarrassment and small mistreatment—for example, when an acquaintance dumps us, fellow workers backbite us, someone falsely accuses us—our uniqueness can feel surprise. Although we know most people experience these injustices in their lives, because we know (believe in) our own goodness, we don't expect to be mistreated as others are.

The gift in these painful little moments of maltreatment is to feel re-united with the human race. We can say to ourselves: "I *can* understand others; I experience what others experience, I feel what others feel, the game of human life that I play is the same game everyone else is floundering through."

We each sometimes do heroic jobs and sometimes make a mess of things and sometimes get our laurels and sometimes get a really bum deal. This doesn't take the pain away when someone mistreats us, but accepting the gift of rejoicing in our common connectedness can give us a little distance from the heartbreak. We can mend much faster by putting it into perspective: "That's life. Wow, I forgot; I forgot that life is risky, and that laws and principles are guidelines but people are real and unpredictable. I forgot that bad things don't happen only to bad people. Now I remember that other suffering people may be good, too. We all get broken unfairly now and then, and we need to give each other a hand. . . ."

Feeling our connectedness, our ordinariness, can give us the courage to accept how we're unique: we're never *too* different. We are each uniquely different from others and yet always very common. Ironically, part of our commonness is that every one of us is unique and afraid of our uniqueness. In accepting how we're different from others, we can also grow in respect for everyone else's individuality. And we might even be able to sympathize with those who are still hiding in the crowd, those afraid of being the special persons they are. We know that fear, too.

We probably all feel intimidated by or alienated from different types of people we meet. We feel in awe of some people and feel we can't relate at all to others. When a little heartbreak puts us in balance again with both our commonness and uniqueness, it also connects us as equals to all these people whom we've either idolized or looked down upon. We can now say to ourselves, "Because of my uniqueness, no one in the world is better than I; but because of my commonness, I am not better than anyone else."

The ability to take a deep breath and laugh at one's self is what enables these two opposing parts of ourselves to make sense together. These painful times when we feel our commonness can enrich and strengthen our uniqueness through the bridge of humor. We might look at our situation differently if we thought of the person who hurt us as a court jester and ourselves as queens or kings:

> It was one of the redeeming features of ancient and medieval monarchies to have recognized that every king needs a court jester, a part of whose function it is not only to make the king laugh but to make him laugh at himself. . . .This not only reveals what he is, and prevents him from pretending to be what he is not, but allows him to be what he really is: A person like everyone else who participates with all his subjects in the frailities and follies of the human condition. . . .Through the court fool the king preserves both his sanity and his humanity.[3]

My pain looks very common,
many others have my pain.
Generic pain;
all day long the soap operas tell my story.
So . . . I'm initiated now,
    welcomed into the hoi polloi,
    finally a real human being.
I thought I was above these common experiences:
rejection, petty gossip, misjudgement, heartbreak.
My Uniqueness feels offended.
But someone inside me laughs at her—
she is so funny, my Uniqueness.
She specializes in our specialness.
But she forgets that we have commonness.
Here we are with millions of others;
all in the same moment we feel the same pain.
We all have broken hearts,
we've all been misunderstood,
    rejected,
    under-appreciated.
My pain is soothed by the company of others.
My laughing self says,
"This, too, shall pass.
We shall all survive. . . ."

26

Truly Little Pain

I absolutely refuse to allow anything or anybody that touches my life to take away my inner poise or tranquility or peace of mind. I know that life will bring many challenges, but I refuse to allow anything to have power over me.

—Author Unknown

FOR MANY YEARS WE IN THE CHICAGO AREA HAVE BEEN blessed with a love advocate, a sprite of sunshine and warmth. For forty-two years, ever since Walter Darson hit bottom, pulled himself out of the gutter, and started up a different path, he has been teaching people about love.

When I want to feel sorry for myself, Walter's story silences me. It starts back in childhood with neglect, abuse, and abandonment—situations no child can handle and too many children experience. Perhaps early crucifixion can lead to early resurrection. By twenty-two Walter had hit bottom. Then Grace stepped in and offered him a second chance. He took it. Little by little the new path opened before him, and he went with it. He turned his face away from bitterness. He was alone in the world and lonely, so he decided to *give* love in order to have it in his life. And he rejected his old escapes from pain and learned how to find joy and pleasure in other ways.

Walter can feel ecstasy when finding a flower in a hidden place. He focuses on the sun peeping through rather than the clouds interfering. A phone call from a friend is not just "pleasant": he allows himself total joy over every good occasion. If his roof is leaking and he has no money, he patiently empties the pails while thinking about the great phone conversation with the friend. He's a dancer, because his soul is alive and ready to dance. He's a hugger, because his heart and arms are open. Countless people thank Walter for his guidance and his affirmation of us.

I learned from Walter Darson that happiness was a choice! I had thought that if it was cloudy I *had* to feel down, and that if there was something to worry about I had to worry about it. In him I saw someone with real reasons to be unhappy who was choosing to be happy. There is always as much reason to face one direction as the other; what we will focus on is our choice. There is always something lovely to see, to do, to remember.

We all know the riddle: If a tree falls in a forest and no one is there to hear it fall, is there any sound?

Is pain a matter of attention? If we don't feed it with attention, will it stay very small? Will it exist at all?

If pain is a feedback system, it could be dangerous to ignore it. But why not treat it like an irritating co-worker: deal with it as best you can, change the situation if possible, and then smile and put up with what cannot be changed. You can say: this person/this pain is not going to rob me of joy and peace; I will not give it any more power than I must.

My pain is truly very little.
There is so much non-pain in my life!
There is so much sunshine,
so many good and wonderful people,
so many delightful things to see
or touch or hear or smell or taste,
so many interesting challenges,
new things to learn and do. . . .
The world is endlessly full of delightful elements.

My pain is small beside my blessings.
Sometimes I neglect my pain entirely:
becoming so absorbed in some wonderful happening
I forget my poor pain.

I wonder where it goes when I forget it.
Does it exist at all
if I don't affirm it?

27

Fear and Courage

You are at the mercy of your emotions only when you fear them. . . . Fear, faced and felt with its bodily sensations and the thoughts that go along with it, will automatically bring about its own state of resolution.

—SETH

THE WIZARD OF OZ, THAT GREAT GRANTOR OF DEEP LONG-ings, taught me a valuable lesson. After years of seeing this movie over and over I finally realized that when the wizard gave the lion a badge of courage, the tin man a symbol of his heart, and the scarecrow a diploma, he was not giving them what they longed for: he was acknowledging what they already had but didn't realize. In the story, whenever an idea was needed or a decision had to be made, it was the scarecrow who came up with the good idea; he already had a brain but had accepted the idea that he was "stupid." The tin man ob-viously had a heart all along; he cried frequently when things touched him. And then there was the lion who thought he was a coward because he couldn't stop trembling when he was afraid—but he would not let anyone attack or hurt Dorothy if he could prevent it. His problem was that he thought a courageous person would never tremble and shake!

In watching this story I realized what courage is. Courage is not the absence of fear, it is acting freely in the way we choose *while feeling fear.*

A person who feels no fear simply acts in whatever seems a logical way; others might call it courage because of their own fear, but for the non-fearful it's just the thing they do. After driving for some years, most people no longer feel fear when they sit down to drive a car; we drive barely aware that we're driving, and we often enjoy driving as if it were recreation. But all new drivers feel trepidation each time they get into the car, and they're tense and fearful for a couple years. The veteran driver is not exercising courage but is just driving; new drivers are the ones who can feel proud of their courage. But if a young man speeds through traffic because he has no sense yet of the pain and problems in accidents, he's not acting with courage; when an older person speeds through traffic to take someone to a hospital she acts with courage: she has the proper fear because she comprehends the danger in what she's doing. The young soldier who goes off to war thinking this is all about being a hero is not acting from courage but from mis-information; the seasoned old soldier who has lost friends in battle understands what he's involved in and must act from courage.

Besides the presence of fear, point of view has much to do with the definition of an act as courageous. Every one of us daily faces situations in which we feel some fear or unsureness or apprehension. Like the lion, our own thoughts may tell us that we "shouldn't" feel fear, and so we think we aren't really courageous. Then we must correct our judgment: emotions are not to be talked away, they just "are"; and when in spite of our fear we get ourselves to act according to our choices,

125

we deserve to pat ourselves on the back. Perhaps no one else knows that we just exercised courage; maybe others wouldn't fear doing what is difficult for us, but other people have their own different challenges. When we know we've mustered courage—taken a first step in a rehabilitation room, confronted a person whom we felt wronged us, tried to do something new, told the truth, or done any small acts that *we* know took a lot of energy—then we should acknowledge to ourselves that we've done a good job. "Good going, Matthews," I say to myself.

So much of our experience of pain has to do with things going on in our heads. Remembering the past and feeling bitterness merely increase our own suffering; "imagination"— the cause of fear—does the same. Imagining what isn't here yet drains energy we need now. We can handle the pain we have now, but we cannot handle past, present, and future pain all at once. For fear is not connected directly with the pain of the moment. The pain of the moment is already here and is hard to bear, but we're doing it. Fear takes this and shoots its power into the future: What if *this* never goes away? What if *this* gets *worse*? What if . . . ? "This" may be terrible; but all Life asks us to handle is only this. Or, as was said on a PBS broadcast on pain, "As pain becomes dominant it seems to say, 'there's nothing more important than this.' When pain takes over completely it ceases to inform but, instead, now interferes."[4] The great challenge in both emotional and physical pain is to refuse to let fear swamp us, to decide instead to keep our heads aware of the whole while attention is being pulled toward a part.

Although I am a Quaker and a pacificist, I must confess I enjoy watching football. Brutal as the game is, what I love is watching courage in action. The game is a drama of concentration on the goal versus worrying about possible hurt. To jump at the ball with total gusto, knowing that when you come down, easily more than 1,000 pounds will pounce upon you—I'm truly awed at this! Watching it gets my own adrenalin going, and I feel inspired to be more courageous in my life. Perhaps this has always been why we love to watch sports events: they are life in theatrical form. We are inspired to play our own little life games with the bravery we see acted by these spunky players.

We can each be heroines and heroes in our small corner of the universe, in the already-created situation that's been given to us. As we refuse to succumb to the temptations of fear, we can create the world closer to the way we want it to be. Each time we expand with courage rather than contract with fear, our own lives and the whole universe expand a little.

Pain doesn't matter anymore.
It's so familiar to me
I scorn it.
It wants to be the center of attention;
it wants me to make a big deal of it.
It wants to intimidate and obscure me.
Well, I will be me; I will not be frightened.
Pain seems bigger than it is
because of this team that supports it,
a team of shadows formed by fear.
A shadow is nothing!
I won't acknowlege the presence of a shadow.
You shadows that go before,
you try to hurt me before Pain has arrived:
Be gone, be gone!
I won't acknowledge the power of a shadow.
I plunge in like a football player:
fear of possible pain
   won't stop me from playing the game.
You shadows that trail behind pain and mock me:
I turn my head; I've already forgotten pain;
I give no more power to it.

We wrestle, just the two of us.
Sometimes I win and sometimes pain wins,
but we are an even match,
the two of us.
I refuse to give power to the shadows
that want to distract me,
these fears that are real
only if I look at them.

V

The Physical System

28

My Body Shouts

"I," you say. . . . But greater is . . . your body and its great reason: that does not say "I," but does "I."
—FRIEDRICH NIETZSCHE

ONCE I HAD A TERRIBLE TOOTHACHE. MY ENTIRE JAW ached so much that I couldn't tell if the problem was in an upper or lower tooth. I had thought about the idea that pain was trying to tell me something, and here was a real test of it. While suffering intense physical pain, am I to try to dialogue with it, listen to it? Wait patiently for it to speak? How much easier to run to a dentist and be rid of it!

I remember trying to reassure my nervous parts with positive thoughts: "I'm beginning to understand what my body wants to tell me. I'm hearing the message more and more clearly. Soon I will understand what my pain is saying. I'm ready to change in whatever way my pain wants me to change. . . ." I kept talking to myself in this manner, and thus I kept my anxiety level down and could wait.

My first realization was that the problem must be in the

131

roots, that the pain was deep. And that there must be more than one root hurting. "Roots, my roots are causing me pain," I thought, "the basic elements underlying everything. Like root ideas: perhaps some unhealthy ideas that are hurting me." So I began to say to myself, "I'm ready to change. I'm open to hear new ideas."

Within two days I received five principles to think about. Most came to me as "inspirations," thoughts that were surprising and untypical for me. One or two came to me in dreaming. After I received/accepted these five principles, my toothache went away, and I did not go to a dentist. I've had no work done on that side of my mouth since then.

Here are the new root beliefs I was given:

1. I'm perfectly perfect just as I am.
2. Only do what's fun (or, if it isn't fun, don't do it).
3. The good of the whole is more important than the desires of any of the parts.
4. Leave room for the unexpected.
5. Give up!

These ideas were very foreign to me. Yet there was some level at which I understood them. They were so opposite to my usual thinking that I could feel how healthy they would be for me to try. I began to think them through.

Here are the beliefs I found that I usually held:

1. Because I know many ways I can improve, I judge myself bad when I see that I'm not yet what I can imagine becoming.
2. I must force myself to do the "right" things, dutiful things that others tell me I ought to do. Following my heart would lead to chaos. And enjoying life too much would be immature, sinful, and contrary to duty.

3. I can't help myself. If my palate wants sugar, or any
   other part of me wants something, I have to follow it.
   I believe that I "need" it rather than I "want" it.

4. The unexpected is an interference of some unfriendly
   force in life; the unexpected is unwelcome. The only
   security there is in life comes through control, so any
   unexpected events are interferences in the security I'm
   trying to build for myself by effort and control.

5. Trying harder is the solution: if I just try harder,
   work longer, I can make things work. Relaxing is
   dangerous, because life is a battle. The force of life
   is against us, so our only hope is in our own great
   effort.

These old beliefs were the root cause of a lot of pain. I
thanked my teeth that they had cared for me and had shouted
and forced me to look at my thoughts.

"The body is the Bodhi Tree," says Alan Watts. The Bodhi
Tree was the physical place on earth where Buddha experienced
his great enlightenment. For seven years he had struggled by
the traditional means of self-denial and contemplation to understand life, to find happiness and relief from never-ending
suffering. All his great efforts were futile, but ironically, he
found what he was searching for when he gave up. Watts
describes the moment:

"The evening before his awakening he [Gautama Buddha]
simply 'gave up,' relaxed his ascetic diet, and ate some nourishing food.

"Thereupon he felt at once that a profound change was
coming over him. He sat beneath the tree, vowing never to
rise until he had attained the supreme awakening, and—according to a tradition—sat all through the night until the first

glimpse of the morning star suddenly provoked a state of perfect clarity and understanding . . ."[1]

When Buddha had committed himself to sit quietly in the place where he was, the place itself brought the enlightenment he had sought everywhere else. Sitting in oneness with this particular tree, Gautama Buddha came to experience what life is about.

Our body is our Bodhi Tree. We walk around daily in our place of enlightenment, our temple, while looking all around us, outside of us, for cures to our suffering, for answers to our questions.

Our spiritual guide, our body, is always trying to lead us into wisdom and fuller life. But we run away from our guide. We take a knife and tear out the messages inscribed on the walls of our temple. We take in medicines, pain killers, alcohol, drugs, unneeded food—so many supposed power items—in an attempt to silence the voice of our guide.

We usually treat our body as if we were driving a car: we think we're the driver, and we don't think of it as our guide. We don't pay much attention to its guidance until it shouts to us in pain. Then, not realizing that pain is an invitation, a sign that it's time to grow in some way, all we think of is how to get rid of it. There is only one true and permanent way to get rid of pain, and that is to hear what it has to say and be guided. Stephen Levine described the time when he was in pain and was fortunate enough to find a wise advisor: "I went to one of my teachers to ask how I might get rid of the pain. But instead of buying into my escape mechanisms, he said, 'Don't look for relief, look for the truth!' "[2]

A friend of mine says that all pain is caused by rigidity, by resistance to change. If so, then relaxing should ease our pain. Anything that helps us relax—laughter, music, backrubs, warm soapy baths, walking, dancing, sports, shouting, hugging—any form of re-creation may squeeze us past our resistance to life with very little effort. Stephen Levine adds to this notion that "Surrender is letting go of resistance." What is surrender but relaxing, choosing to trust life when the choice could be either way?

We do not have to fight for health; our body naturally moves towards health. Pain is feedback to the spirit, a door inviting us to greater life. "You are not responsible *for* your illness; you're responsible *to* your illness," adds Levine.[3] When the body has spoken, we must stop and listen. If we try to resist, our pain will get louder: the body will insist on being heard.

Is anything in our world so close and so important to us as our beloved bodies? Although our bodies are "ourselves," they have an independence from our consciousness that feels like a "spouse," a loving but ruthless spouse who will not hesitate to tell us our faults but will continue hounding us till we change.

We are each stuck till death do us part with this truthful, living thing we have each created; each person's body is both self and a mirror of one's self. Like turtles, we are our own homes. Our bodies are our laboratories for learning by experience and libraries as sources of information. Our bodies are our teachers, our gurus, and our daily guides through the unmapped terrain of life. "I limp along in my old pick-up truck," my dream said. It carries me through my adventures, it sputters when it's been abused. Someday I'll say "enough" and leave it behind. But "my old pick-up truck" is the temporary temple I've created for my own enlightenment; it's my vehicle for many adventures and for the expression of my spirit.

O Great Weariness! O Great Agony!
My body cries out in pain and exhaustion.
It stops.
It goes on strike;
It can't respond to more commands.
This feedback system is overloaded;
A fuse blows, and power is cut off.

My body is trying to tell me something.
It says,
"Please give me your attention!
Don't ask me to do anything more.
Don't put anything more into me.
Don't do anything more to me.
Stop pushing me.
And stop trying to help me.
Just *listen to me*.
I can heal myself
if you listen to me, obey me, and don't interfere.
I am both your operating system
    and your feedback system.
You and I are *one system;*
for a moment, don't listen to anyone but me.
Others only guess at what I'm trying to say.
But because you and I are one
you will understand me
if you are open and quiet
and honest.
If you won't understand me

I'll cry louder
till I have no more energy with which to cry out.

You, my spirit, are out of balance.
In some corner of this feedback system
I'm telling you this.
You have created me.
Every nook and corner of me has a particular function for
you.
When I mal-function
my mal-functioning is particular.
Read my lips.
My pain says there is something *particular* you must stop
doing.
Or start doing.
I am a system with limits.
My limits force you to change.
This is your choice:
you may change
or you may destroy me.
My existence is in your hands."

29

My Body Remembers

*When we accept the unacceptable, it has no more power
over us. We can move through and beyond the experience.*
—ELIZABETH WATSON

JOANNE'S LEGS WERE PARALYZED IN AN AUTO ACCIDENT twenty years ago when a drunken driver hit her van. Since then, she has worked part-time and has finished raising her family. She tells me that for twenty years she has *always* been in pain. She cannot move her legs, but they always have an intense burning hurt.

I'm impressed and silent, amazed that she carries on as well as she does. Is there any life-view that can make sense of this endless pain, or is it just another mystery that Fate/God/Nature has whimsically imposed on a helpless creature?

I try to imagine myself "in her shoes." What I feel, then, is my body constantly reminding me of my accident and loss. Like bitterness in the spirit, my body is still remembering with anger. But my body has no mind of its own; *I* am the mind of my body. I, Joanne-the-consciousness, feel the loss still; my body shouts and cries what my spirit would like to cry.

138

I realize again the paradoxical nature of bitterness. Like Wes's sister, Faye, Joanne's loss was great and her anger justified. But she only hurts herself if she bitterly holds on to her anger.

It takes time to adjust to great changes and new boundaries. "We cannot accept the unacceptable in a second," says Baroness Jane Ewart-Biggs.[4] Time doesn't always heal by itself, however; we can resist that healing of time, so sometimes our consciousness must make a *decision* to heal by accepting change. Then the gift in this change can begin to show itself.

Each body is a history book. It's a treasury of a lifetime of living. When it's registering live pain rather than dead scars, something is not a memory yet: we are still experiencing something that only appeared to happen "long ago." Perhaps if we open to the gift our pain wants to give us, it will be able to end its ceaseless cry for attention.

My body remembers.
It remembers an attack,
a loss,
an injustice.
My body is sad
and angry
and indignant.
My body is always in pain;
it is determined to remember something.
My mind thinks that this event is all behind me.
But my constant pain tells me
that in the back of my mind
I'm still remembering.
If only it hadn't happened!
I still wish, I still wish. . . .
I still look back;
pity and anger are yet a little part of me.
I've forgiven and forgotten at least eighty percent;
I've adjusted and gone on by at least eighty percent;
But still this minority part of me
holds a grudge and rebels.
I try to silence it,
but my body hears the cry of the repressed minority.
My body gives voice to it;
My body ceaselessly squeaks and yells
so that I can hear my own truth.

30

Anything Goes Now

*But now I decided—or was I forced?—to explore a chartless
land. . . .*

—OLIVER SACKS

WHEN PAIN IS SMALL WE ARE GIVEN HOPE BY OTHERS.
Medical doctors will first give a long Latin name to our problem; this relieves us from worry, because we think it means
they know what to do. Or the physicians will stop our further
questions by explaining all in this impressive statement: "It's
hereditary." This, too, sounds as if they know something, so
we stop thinking further. We try all the antics and tonics they
prescribe: we jump through hoops, drink repulsive concoc-
tions standing on our heads, we let them cut out anything
they want to take, or stuff garden hoses down our noses. And
after they've exhausted their imaginations while mutilating us,
the problem is still thriving in our system. Where to now?

We've hit bottom. A good physician will say it for us: "I
don't know." We are pushed into the floating place, into mystery. But "I don't know" is a good place to be. Stay there for

141

awhile, trying nothing except to remember that Life is always loving us, no matter how things appear. If we are still alive, it's because Life is still treasuring this form.

The life force has its own momentum. Our pain intensifies and pushes us. There is no familiar guide for us any more, because we've gone beyond what our culture can control. Pain and Grace are carrying us in their arms; they are in control now, and we are moving fast. We can shut our eyes and try to dig our feet into the ground against the flow, or we can take a deep breath, open our eyes, and see where this wild ride is taking us.

We often enjoy wild rides at carnivals and fairs. We let go, knowing we'll come to a safe end. The adventure is exciting. We enjoy moving fast, feeling danger, being scared. So when our pain cries out for resolution, why not let go, relax, and try new things? Why not see where our pain will take us? We have an adventure forming here in our own life; we don't need to watch a movie for excitement. We just need to believe that the adventure is upheld by Love and will be brought to a satisfying conclusion if we don't fear what's happening. Richard Moss challenges us to confront our most life-limiting fear: ". . . to embrace life, the present moment, with the over-whelming pain and fear . . . is . . . beyond most people. . . .We never find out the nature of the love affair that is occurring right now. We are afraid it is not a love affair. This is the fundamental fear. We must pass through this fear. . . ."[5]

Each life raises its unique questions and challenges. We may sometimes seem "odd" to each other for the answers we come up with. But our unique answers flow from the unique questions raised by each life. My own first question was "Why do I have a crooked back?" This is not the same question as that of my friends or neighbors in their particular pains.

142

My medical doctors had thought about the same question, but they couldn't know what it *felt like* to have a crooked back—and what it felt like is data that should be considered when trying to answer the "why"; it can point to the purpose or toward the cause. Nor did the physicians have my memory of the life experiences that preceded this manifestation. Without any evidence, physicians had called it "hereditary," but I had not been born with a crooked back, so surely preceding experiences should be taken seriously. Most of all, lacking pain, they were unable to go far enough in their questioning—not far enough to find answers adequate to the power of the questions. They couldn't get out of the boundaries of the rational mind.

The rational mind wants peace and order; it doesn't want the distractions of emotion or stress. And it cannot even imagine beyond the familiar, because of the discomfort this causes. Pain pushes us beyond the boundaries of the known and comfortable.

Philosophers, theologians, priests, and ministers as well as physicians could write off my questions as "mysteries," unsolved problems, or "eternal questions," because *they* are not in great pain! They're sitting behind desks looking at life (and me) as an object. Pain says that life (and I) are not objects. Life is a *verb;* something is always *happening.* Every event must be responded to, not examined. Questions push for response, and *they have their own directions.* They might even have purposes; questions want to carry us somewhere.

My present pain pushed me to examine my life experience until I realized how I had brought about this physical manifestation of my earlier pain.

Being the oldest of four girls and having no brothers, I was in some ways my father's son, pushed to achieve, to go out and make something of myself in the world, to dream big dreams, and to think that the world was wide open to me. I thought I could do anything I wanted to with my life. Both my parents were proud of any achievements of their daughters "in the world" as opposed to achievements in "womanly" arts and home skills. For five summers I went to a high-powered summer camp for girls "for the training of Christian leaders." Within the camp system one could soar; we were encouraged to try anything, to think of changing the world, to function assertively, and to freely use all our talents. But back in my local school, and in the culture I met in the media (television, movies, even "great literature"), the message I got was that girls were not supposed to soar and achieve. As a matter of fact, the most important thing a girl should do was to attract a man. To do this, one must be less than a man. One must *hold back*. A woman could soar only as long as she stayed behind the men around her.

The mixed messages I was receiving caused stress and confusion. Ingeniously, I stored all my stress and confusion in a hidden place—at the very bottom of my spine. I kept a straight and cheerful face before the world, but "behind my back," where no one could see, where not even I was aware, my body was crying out the truth of the contradictions to which I was trying to respond. I was being pushed and pushing myself while at the same time I was holding myself back. This was reflected precisely in the type of curvature I have—a forward curve, like a sway: pushed forward in the chest, holding back at the base.

I've never found any physicans who could hear the truth about the way I developed a crooked back. It's too far removed from their own experience, too far out for the rational mind alone to grasp.

But pain freed me to find new and wonderful discoveries about the nature of life. I found that I and my body are one, that my experience was not a mystery caused by some fickle power. My pain made sense and had purpose; my crooked back expressed my stressed emotions and guided me toward the truths about the confused messages I was being given. I was led to see that nature has integrity and truthfulness when its language is understood.

Today I still push myself forward while holding back. Bones being living things, I wonder: if I were to stop doing this, might this very large series of living bones move toward its natural curve? I don't know, and I probably never will, because surgeons have grafted it permanently to my pelvis in its crooked state, making improbable its return to its natural state even if I relaxed. But at least I see the unhealthiness of pushing myself and likewise of holding myself back; even if I can't correct this damage, I'll be healthier if I pay attention to what I've learned.

There's more than one cause to any event: the immediate causes of my crooked back were the forces pushing and pulling me. But there's more to say about this than the immediate cause. There are several types of causation. There is, for example, remote causation ("he drank too much at the party"), immediate causation ("he didn't stop at the light"), the goal as "final" causation ("he was in a hurry to get home"), and so on. My crooked back has given me many gifts that might be final causes—positive goals that draw an event to happen. I've referred before to the strange notion I ran across in my reading: that my "eternal soul" might have *chosen* my life situation, with all its limits and possible problems, because they were seen as opportunities to grow in a positive way. This is a hypothesis about the nature of our spirit that is as unprovable to the rational mind as any other, but it certainly turned me around to look at limits in a different way.

It seems to me now that we go through life as if we were each walking down a hallway; some doors are open for us and others are closed. We can focus on the closed doors and waste time imagining the wonderful things behind them, or we can focus on the open doors, *go through them,* and receive the gifts that are waiting for us to claim. Great limitations may be a forceful focusing toward a very particular and strongly desired gift.

To go through a door is to step into the unknown. And we must go through our doors alone. Friends may or may not be with us, may or may not understand all that leads or pushes us. But pain can be trusted to be our guide. Like a biofeedback machine, our pain tells us accurately what is healthy and unhealthy for us. Pain nudges us towards this door and away from that. There is integrity in pain: it is not a punishment but a force that pushes us into expansion. Without a push, we would never take the leap that would allow us to fly free.

My pain is a rocket booster
lifting me into far-out places.
Anything goes now.
All that my culture has to offer
   has not worked for me.
Now I'm free to try the unthinkable.
I make leaps of imagination,
ask impudent questions,
break idols,
form new hypotheses and try them out.
What's to lose? Within my world I was lost already.

All my energy coalesces
and bursts into questions
that the world around me can't answer.
Pain shoves me into unexplored territory.
A reluctant pioneer,
the dark-horse candidate,
   I find myself with the honor of leadership.

I am alone with my questions.

"Unapproved" reads the sign on the fence
that others say to stay behind.
But my unanswered pleas push me on.
The land into which I'm shoved
is feared and forgotten by my civilization.
My society has no maps,
and perhaps no hurrahs.

I find a few footsteps,
a few markers:
I'm not the only person pushed here.

Pain pushes me here,
but I'm not abandoned:
Grace, my merciful guide, awaits my arrival.
She knows the secret way
   to my unique salvation.
I will listen within
for her guiding whisper.
With Her I will walk unafraid
into the unknown and forgotten,
and step by step
we will make a path
for others in pain.

31

Paralyzed

*As a child I loved nothing more than stories of naturalists
and scientific exploration—Darwin on the* Beagle, Bates
on the Amazon. *I had always dreamed that I, too, might
go on such a voyage, travel to and explore far-off places.
And now, I realized, this was neither more nor less than
I had done. There had not, perhaps been much physical
movement; but sitting in a hospital . . . I had travelled as
far, as strangely, as my heart could desire, had seen and
explored a whole new world of thought. . . .*

—OLIVER SACKS

WHAT COULD BE THE GIFT IN TOTAL OR PARTIAL PA-
ralysis?

It is the gift of absolute concentration. When every door is
closed but a person is still alive, there are only two things left
to do: think and feel! These are not bad activities. Being paralyzed is similar to finding one's self in a prison. Physical
immobility forces us to try something new—reflection, and
the open-endedness of time certainly allows for it.

The extremity of this sudden restraint may cause great anguish of spirit. This anguish may be the rocket booster that starts one directly on a new path of exploration. Where can a mind go without its body? What are the unexplored territories inside us?

Dr. Oliver Sacks was thrown by a bull when mountain-climbing and found that his legs were paralyzed; there was no hope that he would ever walk again.[6] He had never been a patient before. How much he learned about healing, both for himself and others, through his observation of himself in his struggle to recover! After his surprising recovery, he became a pioneer in awareness of the relationship between the mind and physical symptoms. He often tries what to traditional neurologists would be far-out ideas, such as using music to heal, but his experience freed and pushed him into far-out explorations that benefit many people.

When we find that our lives have been "determined," we might wonder at the source of this great determination. Who wants what, from this-my-life, with such ambition and determination? Is there somewhere inside us a strong force that directs our life with absolutes? A force saying, "This is what we're going to do now: think and feel into something new. We're going to rise above the limits of our environment and culture and past, whatever it takes."

Limits are not bad in themselves. The other side of great limits is great opportunity. And anguish is not evil in itself; the unseen side of anguish is motivation.

Frozen; my body is frozen.
I cannot move, my body cannot feel.
A vegetable-human.
Now the only feeling I have is in my heart.
My heart feels and feels and feels
and has no voice to cry.
My head thinks and thinks and thinks
And has no voice to express itself.
I can only think and feel.
Is this what the Other wants?
Will there be an end?
The voice inside me says,
"the end will come
when you've thought enough
and felt enough.
and listened enough.

"And the last and greatest truth to learn:
We are not our form.
Form is the house of the spirit.
Spirit is free!
All form is limit, but spirit is free.
And when the house is boarded up,
spirit moves through walls.
The language and science of spirit is new.
Another pioneer! When we've learned what stillness has to teach
then we, the Eternal Movers, will move again."

32

Painful Death

Never the spirit is born;
The spirit will cease to be never,
Never the time when it was not.
End and Beginning are dreams.
Birthless and deathless and changeless
remains the spirit forever.
Death has not touched it at all,
dead though the house of it seems.

—SIOUX PRAYER OF PASSING

WHAT CAN WE DARE TO SAY ABOUT THE BASIC NATURE OF pain? Is it *always* a gift-giver? Is there any situation in which we cannot find some good? What could we say, for example, of someone who dies a slow, painful death?

How hard it is to die, for anyone! It is very difficult for any of us to give up our bodies. The will to live is very strong in us, as it should be. Moreover, we identify ourselves with our bodies and with these personalities we acquire. What *are* we

152

when we're stripped of these? Most of us know nothing else of ourselves but this. It's frightening to have to give them up and jump into an unknown. I've sometimes wondered why it is that most people in the world die in pain. I think it's just this: it often takes a great deal of persuasion to get us to pass on.

My husband had terrible pain in his left arm and shoulder the afternoon before he died. A "specialist" misdiagnosed these obvious symptoms of heart attack and told him to go home and take aspirin. That night he went to sleep in my arms in great pain, and then he died in his sleep. Some days later I dreamt that he explained to me "how" he died. He said that he had left his body in sleep, as we all often do, but because of the terrible pain he could not convince himself to return to his body. He apologized to me; he just couldn't get himself to return.

My grandmother was in a situation quite the opposite. Her spirit seemed ready to die: her mind had turned away from us; she no longer recognized anyone and seemed uninterested in the world. Her spirit seemed to focus not in her body but elsewhere. But there was the body, healthy and normal. She was unable to free herself. She seemed to lack a reason to take the last step. She would have been blessed by the pain that guided my husband on.

Dr. Elizabeth Kübler-Ross says that the last stage of dying is to arrive at a kind of not-caring. One must let go of the people one has loved all these years, let go of the earth and its interests and values and problems and issues, even let go of caring about one's own life—about whether I've "failed" or "succeeded" or anything else.[7]

It's hard enough to do this letting go, this separation, for ourselves, but our loved ones can make it even harder. Many years back, a young trumpeter with throat cancer shared a hospital room with my husband. There was no hope for him, and he was in constant pain. He was from far-away Indiana, so his wife had moved a cot into the hospital room and stayed there with him day and night. They had two sons. The younger, in sixth grade, was going to play his first football game and begged his mother to come home for just one night to see him play. For just one night, the woman left the man she was treasuring. And he died that night.

Could she have kept him alive indefinitely? His body was not rallying. He knew the end was imminent but was simply hanging on in pain for her sake. She could not accept what he had to do and so prolonged his pain.

I do not pass judgement: it is our instinct to hold on to what we love. We do this even in our own dying. We love life, and we hang onto it until pain twists our arms so hard that life is no longer as desirable.

Terrible pain may be the motivator for one to move through the door—into the New and into the Unremembered.

At birth, we struggled with excruciating physical effort to enter this world, and then we lay helpless in our mothers' arms in a new and larger world. At death, our will exerts excruciating effort to save the now-helpless body. The will must finally relax and shed its skin, must give itself into the larger identity, the arms of the Life Force Itself that brought us here and receives us back. Under persuasion, our energy recedes from its form. But even our senses observe that no energy is ever lost; energy only changes form.

"BEYOND FEAR"
BY TOM FORSYTHE

When I am called,
I will go.
I will go back.
I will go back
    Into the stream of life.
Into air, river, bay, ocean,
Into new land,
Into new life.

Cast my ashes
On Barnegat Bay.

Near there I first saw
Ocean, and viewed the
Vastness of this planet.
Near there I heard of the
Bomb of Hiroshima,
And how small we
Humans are.
Near there my mother
Spoke into silence
Of infinite Love.

I will go free of
Distraction. I will
Go back into
Love.

155

33

Rage for Us: Injustice

. . . while birds and warmer weather
are forever moving north,
the cries of those who vanish
might take years to get here.

—CAROLYN FORCHÉ

IN INDIVIDUAL PAIN WE ARE FORCED TO ENCOUNTER A power greater than ourselves and to look at our lives objectively. When whole groups of people suffer the same pain or the same death, how is their experience different? Are the questions that are raised for a group different, or is the voice of pain just louder, more demanding of our attention?

Basically, pain and dying are always felt as individual experiences: we die one by one, even if we're side by side. And every person on earth must die. And most people die in pain. So why does a group tragedy seem especially terrible? Is it a greater injustice to die quickly on a battlefield, in a gas chamber, or before a firing squad than to be eaten slowly by cancer, our bodies violated by tubes, needles, catheters, machines,

156

radiation, and surgical knives in a well-intentioned hospital? Isn't death just death?

We are part of larger communities, larger events. There is not just I and something Other, there is also us/creation and The Other. Experiencing something in a group is a step out of the illusion of the isolated ego. We are one cell in a larger body.

When a whole group of people suffers or dies together, pain does not change, but attention is drawn to something. Large hidden realities become visible. The victims, the villains, and the entire human race are called to loudly by this event: "Look! Look!" Group tragedies offer opportunities for the whole human community to grow.

The vehicle that will carry the gift to the human community is anger. Anger is very important; anger is a gift-bearer. Anger is enormous energy arising in defense of a threatened value. Anger is a communicator. It is the bridge that links the sufferer, the oppressor, and all others called to, when injustice is trying to separate all.

Anger is a force of gigantic energy, and as such it requires gigantic wisdom to guide it. It may feel like trying to ride a wild stallion when we attempt to respond to our angry feelings and to direct this energy in an effective way. Wisdom must be sure that anger reaches out in its proper direction, that those who should hear it do hear it, and that it will not accidentally hurt innocent persons. Wisdom and anger together should reach out as effectively as possible to stop what pain says should stop.

To not express anger is to betray value. What do we protect when we refuse to admit and express our anger? If there is some fear that holds us back, we will be eaten up ourselves by both our fear and our anger. There is no way to not be angry when we are angry. We can only pretend, and so deaden

157

ourselves to our full humanness. Or our anger may turn to bitterness and eat away at our own life force.

Learning how to express anger takes practice; perhaps we will make mistakes as we learn. But our anger is the voice of our pain; we must hear our own anger and then find some adequate way to respond to it. Anger must be heard by us and then by someone else; it wants to be a bridge, and it wants to carry change. It is a divine creative force in us that sees something valued being threatened and rises up to stop this destruction.

The rest of the human community may undergo positive changes in response to their new awareness of a group tragedy, but what about the victims themselves? What can a suffering group receive to redeem its terrible losses?

The opportunity to the survivors of group injustice is to lighten their cultural baggage, an occasion to re-evaluate themselves. It's hard enough for individual people to change, but much harder for whole groups to let go of habits taken on over centuries that may no longer serve well. This is a chance to let go of any unhealthy attitudes, ways of relating to others, traditions that have lost their positive power, beliefs that don't work.

When we go through transformations as individuals, parts of us stay the same, but parts of us change. We cannot hang on to all of the old identity. Time moves on, and experiences change. As individuals learn and grow, so also groups must learn and grow. In some ways, habits and views are harder to see and change in groups than they are in individuals. Group habits have the support of religious ideas, traditions, and group pressure over individual critics. The breaking apart and destruction of a society may be an opportunity for survivors to rejuvenate the spirit of the group.

This is not to say that injustice done against a group of people is good. This is to say that there is something positive the sufferers can take away from this experience. By accepting

158

the gift, we lessen the power of the oppressor, and we change the world situation by strengthening what is within our power to change: our own selves.

Changing whole cultures, large groups of people, takes great force. In group pain, as always, pain is a *ruthless* gift-bearer, cracking open the group for newness to come in. Does this mean that "God has no heart"? Does the Source of Our Life want growth at any expense? Does it have neither mercy nor patience?

Grace cries, but Pain does not. Every pain suffered by a created being reverberates through the nerve system of the Source of Our Lives. The Divine Womb that brought us forth feels our pain, She feels it *as* pain. I know this because I, too, am the source of life, and I cry when others suffer. When my attention is brought to any other life form that's suffering, I feel it myself, I wish I could take the pain away, tears come to my eyes, I hurt. If I feel the pain of others, the Source of All Life must feel it also.

I remember sharing with a friend the awareness that birds grieve. We had each had the experience of realizing that a bird in our yard had lost kin and was grieving. My friend had observed a male bird that had lost both its mate and its young ones; I had observed a mother bird who had lost a fledgling. We had felt pain ourselves as we listened all day to their continuous cries of pain. What could we do? We could not take the birds in our arms; we knew not how to honor their dead. All we could do was "feel with" them in our own awareness.

When a part of a body suffers, the whole body is aware of it. Our pain is felt in the Force that upholds us, it is heard and remembered by the Source of Our Lives. But change of whole societies, which includes free decisions made with understanding, cannot be imposed magically from outside the natural system. Large change must come organically, within the parameters of time and through persuasion by Grace.

Grace will stir up response to her suffering children within the hearts of others. Prophets will be called, leaders raised, knowledge spread, anger stirred, until—in time—each wrong will bring a response. John Woolman tells in his diary of the dream of suffering humanity that came to him and caused him to spend the rest of his life travelling and preaching against slavery. While sick, he "was brought near the gates of death. . . . I saw a mass of matter of a dull, gloomy colour, between the south and east, and was informed that this mass was human beings in as great misery as they could be and live, and that I was mixed in with them and henceforth might not consider myself as a distinct or separate being. . . . I was then carried in spirit to the mines, where poor oppressed people were digging rich treasures for those called Christians. . . ."

When he came to consciousness out of his fever he couldn't speak until "I felt divine power prepare my mouth that I could speak. . . ." As he spoke, he came to understand what the angel in his dream had meant when the angel said "John Woolman is dead." The meaning was the death of his own will, that, as St. Paul had also expressed, Woolman felt the love of God for himself and for all people now living in him through Christ, and that this love was calling him to express the Divine concern and compassion for suffering people.[8]

Of course, John Woolman was a free person. If he had wanted to ignore the calling in his heart he could have, and Divine Love would have sought someone else. The loving Source of Life will eventually find a voice for the cries of the suffering.

Pain does not care about our suffering: it is focused on our growth. But Grace is with us through it all. The Force that brought us slowly to birth and then into growth has declared our value and resents and remembers any attempt to negate us. When someone negates another, Grace cries out forcefully against this. *Grace remembers* genocide, murder, violation. Divine Love will muster force, *through time,* to redeem injustice.

My pain looks very common;
many others have my pain,
and my heart cries out in rage
for all of us.
We will not survive.
The Great Other
in an unfathomable form
will cut us down.
The story is larger than we can understand.
I am a word in this very large story:
the title is "Injustice."
The story has no ending,
it is told over and over again
in thousands of variations
by individuals with great value
and groups with great value.
Many of us will fall
all at once
in different places.
Many of us will fall
at different times
in the same place.
I feel helpless,
My sisters and brothers feel helpless.
The Great Unfathomable Other slashes away
at every belief we hold,
at every assertion we make.
We cry out for mercy and help,
our words come back to us as an empty echo.
Is No One there?

161

And the arms of my spirit reach out like a giant mother.
I want to rock in my arms
all of the aching people of the earth,
every soul cut down by injustice,
   by insensitivity,
     by the de-valuing of the gift of each created life.

Inside me is the Source of Life
Who brought all forth—
in time, with sacrifice, with effort.
She paid the price of each creation,
She knows its worth.
She treasures each small form.

The Great Mother rises up in fury inside me.
I see you cutting down my children!
Cut down my children in this life,
but we will come back
and avenge every beloved fruit of my womb—
in time.
I will be there against the Ruthless Other
in time.
I hear your protest:
your evaluation of creation is known.
We will re-create the world again and again—
in time.
Creation treasures creation,
Creation re-creates creation,
and energy will redeem injustice.

Within time
every wrong shall be righted,
every pain shall be healed by its understanding,
what is separate shall be one and richer.
All the fragments shall come together:

162

one-ness and many-ness—
red and blue and bright yellow
and black and white and verdant green—
all the fragments shall dance in a rich circle of ecstasy
each as itself
   with a place in a sumptuous whole
      in time.

34

What Color Is Pain?

Darkness within darkness.
The gateway to all understanding.

—LAO-TZU

I WAS SEARCHING FOR ADJECTIVES TO DESCRIBE THE Other, this force that we find ourselves up against in pain. The first adjective that came to me was *dark*. The Dark Other sounded right to my westernized ears: ominous, beyond control, uncaring. But I couldn't let myself use it. To equate darkness with evil and negative forces is a bias of our culture. It carries untruth about the nature of light and dark and is an insult to the majority of people on earth, all those who are dark-skinned.

Our bias about light and dark probably flows first out of our separation from nature. If our housing were less fortified, we might be more comfortable with the night. We might go out and sit in the open under the stars or around a campfire. We could just "be" for awhile instead of doing. I have a friend who grew up on a ranch in Wyoming and tells how she and

164

her family recognized and enjoyed the sounds of the night. They delighted in the sounds of animals, night birds, and insects, in watching the stars move across the sky and the awesome changes of the moon.

If we accustomed ourselves more to the dark we would learn to use senses other than our eyes. And we would turn off our analytical minds for awhile to wait quietly in inactivity and hear our intuitions.

What we like to do in western "civilization" is to think with our analytical minds, to make the world into an object that we can take apart and observe. The dark does not lend itself to analyzing life as an object. The dark invites us to engage in relationships, and to think philosophically, and to experience wholeness rather than the parts. Science and the study of parts belongs to day.

There is one very important way in which pain and the darkness of night are alike:

Pain silences logic
    and evades analysis.
It speaks only one word: *"Listen!"*

But this elusive avoidance of analysis is a gift. It is the gift of freeing us from the limits of logic and opening us through intuition into the unlimited guidance of Grace.

The darkness of Pain is the door itself
that opens to the sunrise of a truly new day
in a truly new world. . . .

165

Pay attention.

Pain is dark,
"the Dark Other."
This sounds right
you say.

You aren't watching at all.
You didn't see me in the redness of rage?
Did you notice my orange face,
my rosy pink face,
my terrifying white face?

Surely you saw me in absence of color—
the pallor of uncoming death?
Now do you remember? You saw my yellow face
in sickness, disease,
when I was eating up your friend from inside.
You didn't see my rosy pink face, as you were wearing it
when you "could have died of embarrassment."
But everyone else saw me, Pain, on your face.

I tell you, my face is orange as nausea,
chartreuse as shock,
blue as despair,
   blue as the ocean that drowns.

My face is white as the dead in the graveyard,
and white as the creeping fog
that slowly wraps around your legs,

166

that closes in around you;
I am the whiteness of confusion, fear, entrapment.

I am the brown of the earth
    that ate the village in the mudslide.
I am the purple of a penis
    separated from its heart.

I am the blinding white light of a nuclear bomb
eating and killing and melting every created thing.
I reach out my terrible white many-arms
and eat up the small and the large, the old and the young,
the hard and the soft, the evil and the innocent—
I am the white light that eats up all creation
indiscriminately.

Oh yes, I may creep up on you in the dark.
But pay attention!
Notice the true nature of night.
The day is turmoil,
the dark is peace,
The day is struggle,
the dark is rest.
In the day one sees clearly the Immediate,
but one cannot see Far.
The Immediate is unclear in the dark,
but one sees the *Whole Universe*.

Therefore,
one sees Reality in the Dark only. . . .

I am the Dark Other,

and the White Other,
and the Red Other,

here to save you
through pain.
Take my blessing.

35

Healing

The question "Where might we find our healing?" expanded. It was the healing of a lifetime. The healing we each took birth for.

—Stephen Levine

HEALING AND BREAKING IS PART OF THE WAY WE CREATE the world, along with choosing/valuing. When we feel out of balance in our bodies or spirits we feel pain, and we long for equilibrium. Healing is whole-making; we search for something lacking that will bring us back to balance and wholeness.

We needn't feel guilty about being out of balance. Any act of trying something new, reaching out, expanding, is an act of leaving stability. Trying something new is good! Reaching out for the new is creative.

But after we've reached out, we feel the strain from reaching and from being out of balance for too long. We search for something else to balance the new and to integrate it with the old and familiar. In other words, we feel broken and look for healing. Then, after being in balance again for awhile, we feel

169

bored! Balance is not dynamic: when in balance we tend to fall into a comfortable mold. Although reaching out is exhausting, it's also exciting. Our lives are like the waves, expanding up and out with exuberance and then settling back into stability, only to repeat the dance over and over and over. Healing brings us into stability.

We are always searching for the story that makes sense of the experiences we've been given. When we find the story that pulls together all the parts of this life, the parts feel like a whole. The story has healed their disjointedness.

We sometimes explore the parts first as parts; then we must integrate them into a whole. A boy must become a man. But then he must find the feminine inside himself and no longer rely outside himself for that part; then he will be a whole person. A girl must be a woman. But eventually she must feel the masculine inside her and let it live, and so she will finally become a real person. The goal of all of us is to become a whole and real person. We can become this only by first being either a man or a woman. But to stop at that is to miss our wholeness. We must reach out of our limits and heal our weak, undeveloped sides. This healing and growth makes us a person.

My mother lives inside me. My father lives inside me, too. Not in memories, but embedded deep in my personality, my attitudes, my habits. I most notice them living here when their ways are not working. But sometimes I see their gifts inside me, too. When their ways are not working, I blame them for my pain. Why do I have to handle what they failed to handle? Because this is the way the game is played, this is "history." Our parents received gifts and problems from their parents and did the best they could to heal the unhealed. What they pass on is the best they have to give. Now it's my turn to try to use and heal the family inheritance, both the gifts and the challenges.

Each of us with our sisters and brothers all had to find

personalities separate from each other, so we developed some parts of ourselves and let them do the others. Often I've said, "I'm not like that; it's my sister you're talking about." To complete ourselves we must embrace the personalities of our sisters and brothers, the undeveloped selves that live inside us. I heal when I embrace my siblings.

The "family diseases," those physical problems that medical doctors say we've "inherited genetically," these are expressions of the total family inheritance. The true inheritance is the family spirit—the attitudes and values, the strengths and weaknesses of character that our parents received from their ancestors and worked with as best they could. Now they pass on to our generation an accumulated "way of life." To heal *any* physical problem, including the dis-ease we carry in our genes, we must look at the spirit.

Possibly, this is this how genetics changes, species adapt, newness emerges. Consciousness inherits, evaluates, and responds. And expands and heals, expands and heals. . . .

Healing of the body alone is not healing. If the body is to stay healed, something must move in the spirit. In the end, however, healing the body is sure to fail someday, because another rule of the game is this: You cannot have this body forever. This body is a vehicle of experience created by an eternal consciousness in order to expand and be creative. The act of healing the body is an act of expanding one's true self.

The problems of the our physical existence are opportunities. We are here to expand and then come into balance, and we will do this over and over, like the energy of waves.

What is happening in the world?

Only one thing is happening in all the world:
The expansion of the universe
　through breaking and healing.
Finding form,
　then breaking out,
　　then healing into balance.
Then stretching out of balance, trying the untried,
then searching frantically for balance,
then falling into form,
then breaking out of form,
healing into balance.

Finding form,
　then breaking out. . . .

Healing is what's going on.
Or, at least, "trying to heal."
Every war is an unwise attempt
to expand or to heal.

Every murder is an unwise attempt to solve a problem.
Every execution of a murderer is an unwise attempt to solve
a problem.
Every death
is the closing of a lifetime of trying to heal.
Every death is the joyful relaxing
　into the Ground of Life
　　by a soul that "tried,"
that grew,

that took what it was given
and tried to integrate it,
to make out of the given
a beautiful story
by healing the broken parts of the life.

As we reflect on our pain
   we imagine a story without this pain.
We move to heal the bad parts
and so create a better world.
All creation expands by reflecting on its pain.

My wound becomes a place of power.
My wound has purpose,
when from my own woundedness
I feel the wound in another
and give my effort to help heal another;
the balm of "meaning" heals my own wound,
I have a place in the Whole.
My power is doubled by use and by connectedness.
And the universe is warmer, deeper, brighter, richer
   through love.
Only one thing is happening in the whole universe:
expansion and enrichment
   through forming, breaking, healing.

36

What Does It Mean to Be "Safe"?

She who is centered in the Tao
can go where she wishes, without danger.
She perceives the universal harmony,
even amid great pain,
because she has found peace in her heart.
                    —THE TAO TE CHING OF LAO-TZU

IF WE THINK OF SAFETY AS AVOIDING PAIN OR DEATH, we set ourselves up for seeking the impossible. There is no physical or emotional safety. If the purpose of living is growth through finding forms, breaking out of molds, and healing into balance, we will always feel some stress or pain when we expand into the new and unknown. In other words, we cannot avoid at least some discomfort in life. But we have a natural desire to avoid pain. Is there anything we can do to minimize the amount of pain we experience? Can we increase our safety from pain?

"Life is a daring adventure or nothing at all,"[9] said Helen Keller, who had neither sight nor hearing and yet went daily out into the world to be part of life. The desire for safety didn't keep her from living life to the fullest. She appeared defenseless, but she was not, because she learned to trust her inner senses more than her outer senses.

"There is no safe place in the world. The only safety is inside ourselves," says my friend, Hilde Weiler, who as a child was a refugee in World War II.

We have more resources than we use. Inside us we have two halves to our brains; each faces a different direction. The left brain faces out; with it we maneuver through the physical world. The right brain faces in; with that part we are connected to our Source and to each other; through the right brain we are part of larger wholes we cannot see. Can any cell in the skin see the whole body or understand its purposes? No. Yet cells can go "right" or "wrong" in terms of the purposes of the body. Cells can feel pain when they've lost their coordination with the goal of the whole.

It's through our intuitions, the senses of the right brain, that we stay connected with The Energy that brought us into existence. Intuitions are sometimes called "feelings," but they are not the same as emotions, which are also called "feelings," nor are they like the physical sensations we "feel." Emotions give us feedback in our interactions with the world. Our bodily feelings give us feedback about the world outside us or about our own emotions that we're failing to notice. Emotions that are ignored lodge themselves in some part of the body to shout to us.

Intuitions connect us inwardly. These "feelings" are like a telephone wire to our source; they connect all of us naturally to information beyond what our own experience knows. The object of intuitions is the world outside ourselves, but what we "feel" here is wisdom larger than our limited point of view.

175

We are part of bigger events, and the whole knows more than does any of the parts. But any part has access to the whole. We are safest when we trust our larger knowing.

The physical senses and the left brain are near-sighted: they see well close around them, but they can see only the exterior of things. Our inner senses are far-sighted, and they touch inner causes and movements.

Instead of talking about our physical senses and our intuitions, we could as well speak of the eyes of the body and the eyes of the spirit. If we maneuver through life with the eyes of the spirit, miracles can happen because we will be receptive to Grace, divine creativity working in our particular lives. The eyes of the body recognize neither Grace nor the existence of non-physical energy sources. The eyes of the body deal only with the exterior of things.

We are loved and treasured and upheld by the Source of Our Life, no matter how scary the events around us may look. We can choose to view the events we're in from a near-sighted or a far-sighted point of view. George Fox describes the confidence of the far-sighted: "And though ye have not a foot of ground to stand upon, yet ye have the power of God to skip and leap in if you are standing in that which is your life that is everlasting."[10]

"Everlasting life" to George Fox was not something to look forward to: one could step in or out of it anytime one wants. He didn't think of it as a state of grace recovered after a Fall, but as a natural state of confidence into which everyone is born. We are all born in love, we are treasured and guided, even through difficult situations.

Just as every part of a body has its own functions and experiences, so each of us is here for unique purposes. And the Source of Our Life did not set us up for failure. Like an acorn that has all it needs inside it to become an oak tree, the original plan for our life includes all that we need to complete our journey. We are a dream being lived out; we are an experience in expanding and creating that was longed for by the energy that brought us forth.

The universe rejoices when we are pursuing our original purpose. When we are living out the dream that is the blueprint inside us, All-The-Power-In-The-Universe cheers us on, pulls strings for us, lays out the carpet for us. We cannot see the carpet, and so we feel afraid. But we must believe the path is there and find the courage to walk it. Step by step, we "feel" our way forward.

As long as we are alive we are being upheld. (This does not mean that dying is a failure: dying is simply a change of form.) As long as we are alive, the Source of Our Life, whatever It is, is treasuring this form, holding us in existence: We are wanted. We don't have to know why we're wanted; the fact that we're alive tells us that Whatever brought us here is still upholding our efforts. It took great energy to bring us into existence, and it takes great energy to keep us going. For whatever reason, this life I'm trying to live is treasured.

To say that we are upheld does not mean that nothing painful will happen, nor that every challenge we face will turn out successful in the eyes of the world, or even in our own judgement. Witness Jesus on the cross: "My God, my God, why have You forsaken me?" This example grips us because it speaks for all of us: nothing is guaranteed; *there is no safety from pain.* And there are times when our judgement cannot understand where Pain is carrying us. Our judgement must relax into the arms of Life, even when the face that Life is showing us is death.

The endeavors of life are fleeting. They are adventures— scary, difficult, fun, satisfying, or unsatisfying. A friend, Tom Martish, tells me that we need only enough security to continue the adventure. The outcome of the physical adventures is less important than where our spirit is carried. We are here to learn and grow and create, and we are guided and treasured as we step out and do our growing and creating.

Walking a tightrope over a canyon
I am safe.
Jumping from an airplane,
trusting my parachute will open,
I am safe.
In front of shouting crowds
throwing eggs at me,
I am safe.
Walking carefully in the fog,
dragging through the sucking muck,
climbing the mountain path in darkness—
if I have to do these things,
I am safe.
Not because walking a tightrope over a canyon
is a safe thing to do.
But if my Life Source brings me here,
if I'm alive and not dead,
then my Life Source is upholding me
and walking across the canyon with me.
This is what "We" want to do!?

As long as I walk with my Source
I am safe.
Balanced between my four eyes—
two eyes looking outward,
two eyes looking inward—
I walk where my Source Force leads me.
I do not have to understand.
I do not have to see the path I'm on.

Step by step, moment by moment,
I ask: are we together?

Where are we now?
Right here. Let me take this solid step.
Then I can feel where the next step must be.

I'm not even safe from falling.
But if I and my Source Force fall together,
I will land at a safe place.

Walking a tightrope
blindfolded in the dark
across a place that feels "dangerous,"
I reach inside to be sure my Guide is there.
If I'm alone, if the Guide is absent,
I'm *truly* in danger.
Stop! Go back,
find where I left my inner Guide.
Stay with The Beloved Force.

I steer the vehicle,
and Grace tells me directions.
"This is crazy!" I shout.
Grace says, "Trust me."
I check again that Grace is there
and knees trembling, tail curled under,
I go forward into craziness.

Monsters bow down as we pass.
Heavy, guarded gates open at my touch.
Warriors stop to carry me.
If I had chosen danger without my Source Force
these would have been roaring monsters, closed gates,
    warriors against me.
But Grace commands all.
When I go forward as the pet of Grace
the monsters show their smiley face;
I, with pounding heart and trembling legs,
am safe.

179

37

The Pain of My Loved Ones

I like to see happiness and to see happy people, especially happy children. I hope they may grow up happy also, but if I had to choose, I would rather see them brave.
—ALAN PATON

AS I WAS GROWING UP I THOUGHT IT WAS ALRIGHT TO share only good news with my parents. They were so happy over good news— good grades, honors, invitations, and so on. In the illogical thinking of a child I deduced that (1) they depended on me for their happiness, and (2) I would make them sad if I shared any "bad news"—my failures, sadnesses, worries, hurts.

As I look back I realize how hard it was to have no one with whom I could share the difficult parts of life. Adults find support talking with a spouse or friends or counselors, or even in books. For children, adults would be the ones who could help them find words for their pains and help them have perspective on their experiences. Too often, parents aren't available and open enough when children need to talk about difficult subjects.

As my children were growing up I encouraged them to share with me anything that was happening. I have to admit it was often painful. In the limited view of children they might draw dire pictures: "*No one* in the whole world likes me." "Someone invited *everyone* to the birthday party but me." "Everyone was laughing at me." Usually I could do nothing to change these situations, and the child's sadness fell over my heart. Yet the child went away lighter. My willingness to listen had silently said: "This is not unmentionable or unthinkable, so it's not unbearable or abnormal."

Sometimes the children told me things that shocked or worried me. Then I would try to keep my emotions quiet so that I could hear their reasonings and so that they wouldn't feel defensive when I shared my view. We cannot force our loved ones to walk their paths by our rules. Furthermore, they'll hear our views better if we respect their freedom to make their own lives.

Accepting our loved ones as different and separate from us is one of the greatest tests of true love. It's easy to love others when they do and think in the same way we do. Can we love *all* of them, including those ways in which they choose to be different from us? A wise friend of mine, Joey Rodger, expressed our anguish when she said: "We all want to be known and loved, and we fear that if we're known we won't be loved and that in order to be loved we can't be known. . . ." Who can cause us more pain than those who claim to love us but won't love what we are?

If we try to encourage others to change particular parts of themselves, it must be clearly established first that we embrace them unconditionally, that we love the whole of them while criticizing a part. Many years ago, when my husband and I were dating, we argued a great deal. He would ask me to come close to him and hold his hand while we argued! This felt contrary to the cantankerous feelings I had toward him, but he explained that he wanted to feel that, although we disagreed on a particular topic, we were on the same side of the fence. Too often the love that unites us is not clearly established when we try to persuade our loved ones to change their minds or mend their ways. They feel unfriendly pressure rather than loving concern.

I would rather my children tell me all than have them bear the unbearable alone. I don't have to solve their problems. They have their own relationship with Life and Grace, and I have confidence that they are loved and guided by the Source of Their Lives.

All this is as true, of course, of adults whom we love—our spouses, our parents, beloved relatives, and friends. If you've ever accepted the awkward condolences that people offer when you've lost a loved one, you know what a life-giving act is the simple affirmation of caring. No one can bear my pain except me, and I cannot bear another's pain. But we can hold each other up when we're weary and encourage each other on our paths. This is love given with respect.

The way to help our loved ones achieve the most happiness in life is not by protecting them, or pressuring them, or even helping them. The two most important things we can do for our loved ones are to encourage their belief in their own integrity and ability and to nurture their confidence that life supports them.

We can do this in several ways:

- By sharing with them realistic attitudes about life; not sheltering them from truth. There are truths that are hard for all of us to admit but easy for most of us to see; we can point our loved ones in healthy directions, such as "people have to work to get what they want." "Pain will come, and you can survive it." "Death will come, and it will be okay." "We will grow old and weak and feeble, and it's okay." "Not everyone will understand or like you, and it's okay." "We cannot do everything at once." To accept reality ourselves and help our loved ones do the same is a great gift to them.

● By encouraging our loved ones to try things for themselves: to set their own goals, to make their own decisions, and to bear the consequences for those decisions. *It's okay to make mistakes*: this is one of the attitudes that most builds healthy confidence and competence in any of us.

● By expressing our own confidence in their ability to handle their situations. To *show* our worry about another is a statement of "no confidence."

It is in the nature of love to feel pain when a loved one feels pain, or to worry when a loved one seems to us to be in danger. True love takes control of these emotions and chooses to act wisely. We don't want to increase the suffering of those we love by pressuring them when life is already hard and confusing. A supportive, affirming attitude that respects their independence is the most we can do to ease the pain of our loved ones.

There are at least two kinds of pain we feel toward our loved ones: the helpless empathy of watching while undeserved pain comes down on someone we love, and the anger we feel when we think a loved one is really messing up his or her life. In either case, our helplessness can feel like whirlpools of agony in our stomachs or like gigantic erruptions of passionate feelings. A friend of mine has expressed for all of us the passionate eruptions of a caring parent:

183

A Prayer of Rage
by Tom Forsythe

Mother spirit of the earth,
I need your love to hear my pain.
Do not silence me and tell me
My love must wipe out all pain and
Destroy my anger.
                    No!
Hear me rage!
Let the earth shake
(Poseidon and Aries, come!)
With my discomfiture!
Let me not back off
From the truth of my dark feeling.
THIS MUST NOT BE!
My daughter suffers,
And she chose her path
With a troubled mind.
I cannot bear the pain she
And hers will have to endure,
Because she is mine
And I suffer for her
And through her.
And I must live my life.
And do my work
And love my love,
All my loves, not just
My troubled daughter.

184

All Goddesses and mother saints,
Comfort me and receive my tears.
Hold me secure in your love.
Jesus and the father gods and
The crazy tormented pagan gods,
And the marvelous ones, the fighter
And the singer, and the seagod
And the cloud god, and the craftsman,
All the brother gods, and friends,
Men and women, my people,
Hold me in your love now
And cleanse me with your faith:
Prepare me to meet Job and his god,
But not yet—grant me a
Preparing time:
Let me not be programmed by
Such a dissonance as now I feel,
But strengthen in me the breath of
Harmony until it
Can grow
Strong.

You hear me—
I will rest in
Your answering prayer.

I cannot protect my loved ones from pain.
Nor from death.
And no one can protect me.
I cannot avoid pain and my dear ones cannot avoid pain.

I can protect them from some pain
by forbidding them from doing things:
Don't act.
Don't interact.
Don't react.
Don't try anything new.
Don't stand out.
Don't . . . Don't . . . Don't. . . .
Stay in our home/womb
and ~~you'll be happy~~ you won't be hurt.

Pain—and Death—are part of the game.
To be born human
is to accept pain
as one of the guides for the trip.
And death as the transition back.
The football player who doesn't expect pain
has chosen the wrong game.
Better to have been a rose with thorns,
a turtle with shell,
a skunk with smell,
a porcupine.

Rather, my prayer is this:
May you, my dear ones, be wise enough

186

to learn what pain comes to teach you.
May you become more beautiful because of your pain.
Be guided; don't resist learning!

May you, beloved ones, be stronger than your pain.
When its weight feels stronger than you, seek allies!
Seek help, seek advice, seek support!
This is human intelligence:
    to figure out what is needed to deal with the adversary.

And oh, ask me for help!
At least let me cry with you,
even if I can't change things.
I will be a wall for you to lean on
when you're weary in your struggle.

And be there for others, for me,
for anyone who needs help.
The attacker can feel like a giant,
but if we stay together we can manage the challenges.
I do not ask that my loved ones feel no pain;
I pray that they are never conquered by it.

38

Embracing Life, The Whole Bag

"Only if one loves this earth with unbending passion can one release one's sadness," don Juan said. *"A warrior is always joyful because his love is unalterable and his beloved, the earth, embraces him and bestows upon him inconceivable gifts. The sadness belongs only to those who hate the very thing that gives shelter to their beings."*
—CARLOS CASTANEDA

FOR MANY YEARS I OCCASIONALLY HAD WHAT I CALLED "escape dreams," in which I would dream I was trying to escape from different places—concentration camps, prisons, mental institutions—always with the same dilemma: there was no place to escape to; nothing could happen except that I'd get caught again. Trapped, I could not get out.

From what was I trying to escape? I pondered the dreams for years before I recognized what I was running from: *being me!* What I don't want is to be me. What I run away from, in many different ways, is the pain involved in being this particular limited person. Marcia Lynn "Marti" Matthews: oh, anybody but this!

Not only did my night dreams center on escape, but my romantic day dreams centered on being and doing things that I am not and cannot do. Over and over: I don't want to live this life that I am called to live, to be and become the person that I was born. Not the person I was born "to be," as in some goal or dream or ideal, but the whole acorn that I was born *as*.

Why is it so painful to be the person I was born? Why does it feel like a *choice*—as if I could be or not be who I am, as if I have to choose to be me? Why does it take so much effort to be true to myself? Why does it seem to be taking my whole life to become me?

It takes a lot of energy to keep my attention here in this moment and in this body. My spirit wants to dance and soar, to do great things and be bigger than life. But what I intuit is that my path to wholeness and holiness and happiness and power is *through* being this particular little, limited person. The more true to her I can be, the more I will be one with all that's infinite and glorious in the universe. "She" is my path to all that I can imagine.

I've tried to follow the advice of many different "holy teachers," "great spiritual paths"; I've studied religions and philosophies, and I tell you truthfully, the majority of these paths all moved in the same direction as my escape dreams—out of the world, out of the body, out of the flow of life, away from the earth. Think *about* life as an object, not a verb; try to control the flow, kill the ego, subdue the body, avoid pleasure, withdraw from the world, keep a distance from others, feel less: the religions of the world pull us away from creation. "God created the world—and it was bad" is the true belief of most religions and spiritual paths. We are afraid of the challenge of being human; we are afraid to really be what we are—human beings in a world of dirt and changing things and dying things.

What pain! Our pain comes bursting out of us in so many directions; our alienation from our own selves cries out for re-unification.

Marcia Lynn "Marti" Matthews—this is the gift given to me, the great opportunity for which my soul longed. This is my sacred path. I don't need to search for the path of enlightenment; the path is given. All of us are already *on* the path that leads to the highest to which we can possibly aspire.

What is the path to holiness and greatness that's been given? These are the spirit-building challenges assigned us through nature: a constant need for food; for connectedness with others as well as times of separateness; for productive work as well as recreation and rest; for pleasure and delight, which give us joy and energy on our path; for growth and expansion, risk and adventure, problems and challenges, and "meaning"—a place in a larger story and community. These and other elements are what are given by the Source of Life. Pursuing these is what we are called to; this is our path to holiness and fulfillment.

We might find ourselves out of balance—pursuing one need and not our others—but this does not mean the path is evil. This does not mean we should run away from this path. We should simply seek balance.

When it's time for us to be in another world, then we will find ourselves there. Right now, we are called to throw ourselves passionately into being here. And into being someone particular, small as it may feel. "Whatever you do may seem insignificant, but it is very important that you do it," said Mahatma Gandhi, who never founded a "religion" or thought of himself as a spiritual teacher. He lived passionately in the world, and to him there were no lowly people.

To embrace our lives and our selves, the whole bag, is the goal of being alive. It's the path to anything we want. It can take all the courage and effort we can muster to be ourselves and love our lives! But to live fully and to learn how to be our true selves is the highest accomplishment we can possibly reach.

Sonnet: Embracing Me

I wish, I want, I hurt, I fear, I hide.
I hurt enough to stop and watch my pain.
I judge not what I see as bad or shame,
but simply watch what passes here inside.

I love each corner, shadow, hidden place,
I bless each wound and disappointment seen;
I love the fat, the plain, the weak, the mean—
all parts of me I bless with mercy's grace.

"Just this much" is not too hard to do—
to be myself with love and not with fear.
When I embrace myself, hurt disappears
and for this moment I'm O.K. and new.

I stop my hurt: I judge myself no more.
And in my self-embrace I stop the war.

With appreciation to Stephen Levine and Seth

39

I Win!

Blindness is my greatest happiness!
—JACQUES LUSSEYRAN

WE STARTED OUR JOURNEY TOWARD PAIN IN ANGER, asking both accusingly and pleadingly, "Where can love be found in pain?" Now that we've spent time with this unwelcomed guest, does pain look the same? Perhaps at least our pain has more dimensions to it; maybe we see elements in it that we hadn't noticed before.

How do we view *ourselves* now? Are we richer than we thought? Do we have more reason to love ourselves and feel proud of ourselves? Have we come closer to feeling at peace with our lives, that in spite of our limitations and in spite of what feels undesirable, life is worth living? What is the adventure our pain has taken us on? Can we describe yet the treasure that was behind the mask of pain?

Here is a question not for you or me, just a curiosity: What is the long journey that brings a man blinded since the age of

193

eight to say toward the end of his life, "Blindness is my greatest happiness!"[11] Jacques Lusseyran, professor of philosophy and psychology, has described his gifts in detail and with great enthusiasm. He describes, for example, discovering that "the source of light is not in the outer world. . . . The light dwells where life also dwells: within ourselves." For Lusseyran, this was not a metaphor; this was a true light by which he learned to maneuver through the physical world. He discovered the effect of love or hate on his ability to "see" his way around, and he let go of surface judgements and developed an uncanny ability to know people's character without eyesight. His reputation for accurate judgement of character was such that he was assigned the job of interviewing prospective members for a French resistance group in in World War II—a heavy responsibility with hundreds of lives depending on his judgement.

Lusseyran discovered that inner attention could enable a person to "touch" the world without physically touching it. "The shadow of a tree . . . is . . . audible," he said. "The oak, the poplar, the nut tree have their own specific levels of sound. . . . The same is true of a wall or a whole landscape. . . . Finally, even thoughts take on weight and direction." His life was rich, full of treasures he would never have had if he had not been blinded. I truly believe him when he says, "Blindness is my greatest happiness."

But his testimony makes me uneasy. His statement seems to challenge me to ask myself if I could or couldn't say the same: "My crooked back is my greatest joy!" And if I couldn't, why not?

While I was working on this manuscript I had a puzzling dream. It said, "This was life. This was the gift to me—experience. Sacred." On awakening, I thought, "That's nice; that's true. I'm really grateful for the experiences of my life and what they've given me."

Then there was a pause inside me. The dream seemed im-

194

portant, but I couldn't grasp the meat of it. My work was nagging at me, and I wanted to turn my attention toward it. The poetic meditations in this manuscript had come to me spontaneously in a short two months. Now advisors suggested I write an essay to go with each meditation. I needed to find interesting ideas or stories to give background to this mass of poems. Certainly the substance of my life, though valuable to me, would not be interesting to others, as my life was hardly an adventure story.

Or was it? I wrote all kinds of essays and let friends read them. Over and over people preferred the simple stories of what I experienced that led to each new understanding. I was perturbed, because I wanted to write universal ideas that would help others understand their pain, not stories about me. Then a writer-friend, Georgene Wilson, told me that "the more specific you can be, writing from your own experience, the more universal it will be, because people will be able to understand and identify with it."

I was amazed. My experience seemed so little! And it had all occurred mostly inside me, working through my confusions and disappointments as I encountered what seemed like ordinary events.

Across time I kept writing, and over and over with my readers it was the story of my life experience and what I'd learned from it that won out over the abstract and philosophical. The reactions of my friends gradually led me to realize that my life had been richer than I thought. In the quiet interior struggles that no one else had seen, drama had occurred. Inside myself, I had fought courageously against scary demons on foggy battlefields. I had fought injustice in society and stood up for the oppressed (myself); I had changed culture at least slightly. All I had to do was describe in writing these secret battles that had taken place, and describe their outcome and significance for humankind.

"Self-expression always leads to self-expansion," said a quotation I found in my grandmother's handwriting. The gift of my pain was this book. The gift of the book was to enable me to see clearly how special the experiences given to me have been. How much I would have missed without my crooked back! And the book would not have happened without Tom's death.

And being a woman who didn't fit the mold for women? How very rich I feel for all I've experienced because I'm a woman. I've had the double blessing of doing "the things that women do" and knowing how wonderful those experiences are, as well as being able to feel within me the frontiers of all the other wonderful things that women can do, too. There's a part of me that feels I was a lumberjack in another life, a bit of a chauvinist myself. How proud I am to be a woman! How good it feels to learn gentleness, and to feel my feelings freely, to create life, nurse babies at my breast, play with children, and enjoy simple things. What a joy to love freely and feel connected to others as women feel. I'm glad to have been a woman, I'm glad to have experienced the deepening and gifts of grief, and—I'm so glad I have a crooked back.

I bless you, pain, for what you gave to me.
You thought you were hurting me,
but you had no idea how strong I am.
I had no idea how strong I am!
Thank you for opening the door for me;
you led me to a gold mine.
This treasure will make the whole rest of my life easier.
But you may go now;
I found this treasure and I will keep it.
You and your ugly form—I don't need you any more.
You don't believe me?
Come here and I'll kiss your ugly face goodbye.

What! Where are you?
Where's the ugly beast I hated?
Where are you, terrible tormentor?
All I see is a flower—
a sun-filled lily, a beautiful rose, a harmless pansy.
Did I not see you right?
Did you change forms,
or has my eyesight changed?
Here you are smiling at me,
and I can smile back.
Your horny, ugly form has become transparent;
I can see your essence.
You are what you are: another player in my game,
another element in my dream,

A Magi—wise bringer of strange gifts.
I was poor and you brought me wealth;

I was a child and didn't know its worth.
I wanted a toy to play with;
   you brought me exotic wealth befitting an adult.
I thought I belonged in a humble place;
   your attention and your gifts gave me nobility.
O thank you, beautiful gift-giver!
You saw my true self
hiding in a simple form.
You exposed me to the world,
you pointed me out and said
   "This will grow to greatness!
   Watch for what's hidden here inside!"
I didn't even know I was a royal person,
I looked so weak and ordinary.

And you, too, in your ugly form:
who would have guessed you were
my wise and proper benefactor,
my wealthy Patron?
O my gift-giver, as I look back
at my old self, before I knew you—
how poor I would be without you!
What a lot we've gone through together.
You gave yourself to me,
and I have grown.
I am a tall and noble tree now—
a pine, a palm, an oak, a willow.
I'm so happy to feel my beauty.
And now, to me, you are beautiful.
Others call you ugly still,
but in the wisdom of advancing time
my way of judging beauty has changed.
I smile when I think of you.
Perhaps you will pass away from me soon,

198

as everything does.
You will be only a memory to me;
I will let go of you and move on to other adventures.
But you I will always remember—
one of my most treasured companions:
my secret admirer, my guide,
my benefactor, my surprise.

Love came to me in a hidden form,
but I pursued and uncovered it.
I claimed the buried treasure as mine:
I accept Love in *all* its forms.

VI

Moving On

40

Moving On

"I could tell you of my adventure—beginning with this morning," said Alice, "but it's no use going back to yesterday because I was a different person then."
—LEWIS CARROLL

I STARTED THIS LARGE BODY OF THINKING WITH A QUESTION: Where can Love be found in pain? I found pain to be not a negative force but a positive force in nature—one that, while limiting us, focuses us toward some particular growth or change. Pain is not our enemy; the Life Force brings good through both the pleasant and the unpleasant, the awful and the wonderful.

Once we feel that life is solid and nature is trustable even against its appearances, then we can step forth into the world with more confidence. Once we're convinced that our lives exist in a context larger than individuality and longer than birth and death, that there is meaning and purpose to our experiences, then we can let go of fear, unafraid of meeting Life in whatever unfamiliar forms it may come to us. The ground on which we stand is solid. We can dance on it. We can be joyful. If Life is for us, not against us, we can try new things and attempt risky projects.

Although I feel the ground is secure, I ask myself: Where do I want to go now? I look backward and see a path I know. It was full of pain and unhappiness, but this I know, this is familiar. When I look forward, I feel drawn by an outline that's intriguing, puzzling, and scary because it's unfamiliar. I feel as if there's something out there calling me, luring me forward. I want this new life, part of me longs for it, but another part of me tries to hold back still. Why am I afraid of the dream that lures me forward? Perhaps the past was less secure than the future will be! But fears, comfort, guilt, notions of "should" and "shouldn't," logic—these and other chains hold me back to the old and familiar and painful.

It takes so much energy to hold back! My body tightens and freezes and feels "old" as I try to stop myself from running toward this beautiful but unfamiliar future.

I'd like to let go and run forward now that I know that Grace is with me, but how can I make the decisions that must be made without seeing where we're going? What is the basis for knowing the path of Grace?

"Go with whatever is life-giving," a friend quotes me as saying. I said that?! Well, it sounds like good advice; I must know more than I think I know. Choose life, not death; choose whatever gives us more energy, vitality, and joy. This criterion is not hard to use because the body and emotions are our feedback system: they will tell us which path is giving us life and which path is sucking life out of us.

A song that influenced me a great deal some years back went like this:

Born free, as free as the wind blows,
As free as the grass grows,
born free to follow your heart.[1]

204

I felt a large theological opening from this simple song, as if no one had ever suggested that God created us free beings and it was O.K., natural, right to follow the leadings of our hearts. Only human beings have to choose to be natural! Why would we imagine that the Source of Our Life would give inner direction to us and then expect us to oppose that very direction? We are masochistic, and we make life more complicated than it need be. To follow our hearts is healthy; to resist our hearts is to court dis-ease.

The life-giving path feels both familiar and unfamiliar. It's familiar because we've longed for it for so long; it's unfamiliar because we haven't walked this part of our path yet in the way we've passed through "the past."

What will I look and feel like on this new part of my path? At first it feels similiar to "pretending." I move toward being this new person, but I don't know how to do it, I don't know exactly how this new person speaks or conducts herself. Am I a fake? No, because the potential me is real, just unfamiliar. As I relax, her lines, her voice, her lifestyle, her choices and mannerisms will come to me naturally, and then I'll know I'm not pretending: she was really there inside me.

Now I'm moving on, beyond the pain of my past.

Now with long life,
now with everlasting beauty,
I live.
I am traveling,
with my sacred power, I'm traveling.[2]

I rejoice with this Navajo prayer. The time of creating my cup of blessings is finished: now is the time to fill the cup. This is not to say that I won't have challenges or pain still, but the sense of being a victim is passed. Having come to an understanding of the purpose and nature of pain, when I encounter it again I'll be able to act wisely, to listen and dialogue and benefit from it rather than being overwhelmed.

I remember a photograph about traveling that spoke to me of what traveling freely would feel like. It was called "traveling light": a picture of a narrow bridge swinging over a chasm, with Japanese children walking over it, wearing no coats and carrying nothing more than umbrellas. I've always wanted to move freely toward my dreams, but one of my impediments has been carrying too much baggage. Every act of holding onto my past has the negative effect of impeding the wonderful future that is drawing me toward it. "Impede," my dictionary says, is from the Latin *impedire*: to entangle the foot; to stop in progress, to stop one from walking on. Impedimenta: encumbrances; baggage. I try to fly forward, still carrying loads of souvenirs, memories, clothes that don't fit, a self-image that's constricting, relationships that are no longer life-giving, habits that hold me back from being all that I could be. If only I could release my tight hold on everything in my life, so that anything could be taken away from me that isn't a part of my best and most current self, then there would be room for whatever new and wonderful things want to happen in my life. This is my commitment; this is the direction of my effort, to make space for the energy of Grace to move me freely.

For many years I've had in my mind an image that the Source of My Life is a fox. The Light within me sometimes changes directions so quickly that it takes my breath away. Keeping up with the Fox is a challenge: one must be supple and quick and free; one's ideas must stay flexible and open for the unexpected. If one gets too far behind the changes of the Fox, then the merry chase will fade to an end: no Fox, no direction, no motivation, no energy; the life goes out of this particular chase. When we feel inside us that we're being asked to change again or to let go of the past and move on, we'd better relax into the forward movement, lest we find ourselves separated momentarily from our Life Force. That would be a time of despair and might necessitate an ending and new beginning.

"How much shall I be changed, before I am changed!" asked John Donne incredulously. We often long for a finished state, when we can rest forever. Sometimes as I pass cemeteries I think, "Ah, eternal rest. Someday I can just rest!" But it appears to me that this is not the nature of living things. At any moment we are all that we can be, and so we are perfect all the time—yet we will always expand more. Grace is always wanting to increase our joy, so there will never be an ending to our growing and changing. We will never be separated from our Source, as we might lose track of a fox. But our living Source will always be creating us, loving us by expanding us and so increasing our joy.

Letting go,
moving on,
not clinging to what I think I am.
Passing through what I am
to become the forward shadow
that the eye of my soul sees.
I know the outline of the tomorrow me;
Do I have the courage to fall into it?
The outline will catch me,
it's made of solid earth;
what I am drawn toward
is upheld
by the Life Force
that created me originally.
It moves me on, the Life Force,
It knows where we are going,
It has planned a safe course;
It pushes me
and pulls me toward completion.
All I must do is relax
and let the-already-experienced pass behind
and let the magic happen.
If I tense
and cling to what's familiar,
if I hold on to the old
rather than passing through my identities,
if I get stuck
in an identity that is no longer upheld
by my Life Force,

then my shell will die.
The Life Force will move on
   and expand and grow
   with or without this form.
It doesn't need any particular form,
   and it will not be obstructed.
When the irresistable Force
meets the immovable object
It just leaves the immovable object behind
   without its Force.
I love this form.
I will relax
and let the newness happen.
I will walk into the shadow
   that makes my path;
I'll experience the energy that's waiting there,
and the solidness,
and the delightful surprise,
the joy of being all that is in me,
the embrace of idea and experience
   that doubles power.

41

Psalm for a New Morning

There are no atheists in the foxholes.
—COMMON KNOWLEDGE

NO MATTER HOW MUCH WE MIGHT RESIST THE IDEA OF "praying," great pain often squeezes out of us some plea for help from the universe. Dis-ease puts us in relationship with mystery, and to stand in awe and respect toward mystery is what prayer is.

We may send our cry for help on the four winds "to whomever it may concern," or we may have a specific language and image for the Source of All That Is. Often we fall back on words we learned as children. We may feel embarrassed to try to pray, partly because we've been taught that adults should be self-sufficient and not need help from anyone, and partly because these prayers from our childhood are children's prayers. "When I was a child, I spoke as a child," said Paul of Tarsus. For me, the religious beliefs I was taught as a child upheld me well for a long way through life. But there came a point where I sensed that I'd reached the border: these beliefs

210

were now a fence holding me back rather than a support to my growth. I fought against the fence, and Grace led me step by step toward an opening. Then when I'd suffered enough and couldn't stand it any longer, I did as the divers must do and went calmly through the one and only opening I could find.

And there I was—finally at peace, at home, in a new open place with plenty of room to grow. Grace continued to guide me on as I found horizons of understanding that challenged and fed my spirit, and life continued to grow in me.

But the prayers of my childhood did not express the faith of my adult life. I loved many of those prayers, but in particular I could no longer imagine the Source of Life as a "lord." Not only was this an absolutely masculine form of address, it was a type of relationship with the Source of Life that I no longer believed in.

I no longer believed that the Source of Life is complete and without need, that we are nothing, powerless, or full of sin. To me, the Source of Life is sufficient and awesome but also always expanding and changing, affected by us, changed by creation. We are not nothing: the Source of Life longs for us as an expectant mother longs to see this life she's creating be born and grow and flourish and be all that it can be. We are not powerless: the Source of Life waits as a father for the delight of seeing a child's accomplishments, to be enriched by his child's interesting ideas and to see his child be creative and powerful. While for many people addressing the Source of Life as "lord" may be a reverent expression of awe, the relationship to a lord holds the trap of negating our power and dignity, and so absolves us of responsibility. We have power: We affect creation and we affect God. And we are not full of sin: we try ideas and make mistakes, we change our paths and grow. These are the beliefs in which I now stand in the world.

Of all the prayers I learned earlier in life, the one I loved the most was the biblical Canticle of the three children in the fiery furnace, found in the Book of Daniel:

> . . . Sun and moon, bless the Lord: praise and exalt him above all forever.
> Stars of heaven, bless the lord: praise and exalt him above all forever.
> Fire and hail, bless the Lord: . . . Snow and sleet, bless the Lord: . . . Light and darkness, . . . Lightning and storm clouds, . . . Mountains and hills, . . . all things that spring up in the earth . . . seas and rivers . . . whales and dolphins . . . birds of the air, bless the Lord, praise and exalt him above all forever.[3]

This ecstatic prayer of praise for the Source of Life in creation goes on and on.

Because nature is always a church to me, this prayer felt as if it affirmed that creation is good, not fallen, and a blessing no matter the moments of pain, and that the Source of Life is present here, not off in some heavenly place. What a loss that I just could not say this prayer anymore!

One summer morning I sat in my back yard in the shadow of a loving tree whose presence often created a chapel for me. My heart was full as I watched the sunlight dance between the shadows, saw the dew on the grass, and heard the birds and crickets singing their summer morning songs all around me. I longed to say a prayer, both of praise and out of my need to remember that I'm supported in life. So I asked for a prayer; I asked for new words that would both express and lift up my soul. And Grace responded. I share here this prayer, which came first for my own needs, and as much for anyone else who loves the old psalms but is moving on and needs a new psalm for the occasion; I call this a Psalm for a New Morning.

O joyful sounds of crickets and tree toads, praise Life.
O gentle breeze, kiss all Life for me.
O morning sunshine, penetrate each far corner of our darkness.
O blue sky, enfold with your love every person in this world.

O light clouds hurrying by, take away with you all the dead weight we carry.

O birds of the air who bring joy to our souls, come close and teach us the secrets of flying. Lift up our hearts and teach them the trust that will enable us, too, to soar.

O worms in the earth, roots of trees and plants, all you life hidden in the earth, reach down, find and bring us nourishment when our souls feel parched and barren.

O you millions of beautiful trees in our world, teach us how to be still. O loving arms and reaching shadows of trees, pull us into your presence on the edge of time where the eternal view is possible.

O you people of the earth, neighbors and strangers, lovers and challengers, sisters and brothers to me all, I embrace you with passionate love. I honor you, expressions of the glorious Source of All Life. I will try with all my effort to bless you with my blessing, and I humbly await and accept with open arms the blessings you bring to me.

O Fertility from which we are born,

O Fire and Desire that cause me to be,

213

O Love that surrounds us,

O Longing that needs me,

O Awesome Mystery,

the body of my spirit bows before You.

The many and long arms of my spirit reach out across
space;
I love and treasure each manifestation of You.

I do not fear You, Life, in whatever form You appear to
me.

The deep well in my soul awaits with longing,
with confidence,
with surprise and without surprise,
all the gifts You will bring to me.

I will look for Your face in all forms.

You are the source of the river that flows;
You are the water itself, and I am the river
with a name and a form.
You know from the beginning whither our direction,
    what desire is our goal.
My desire is to stay one with Your desire,
    to be all that You dreamed of when You burst forth as
    me.

I let go all the fears of my spirit;
I allow my body to relax in Your all-wise and all-powerful
love.
I am upheld in my life, all that I need is available to me.

I choose to keep myself one with this Solid Ground of my life.
I am loved, I am safe.

Alleluia,
Aho![4]

On the Language Used in this Book

The Tao gives birth to all beings,
nourishes them, maintains them,
cares for them, comforts them, protects them,
takes them back to itself,
creating without possessing,
acting without expecting,
guiding without interfering.
That is why love of the Tao
is in the nature of things.
    —THE TAO TE CHING OF LAO-TZU #51

MOST PEOPLE REFER TO THE SOURCE OF LIFE AS "GOD;" I refer to it as the Source of Life. Because creation is all both female and male or else has no sex at all, so the Source of Life must be both female and male and also beyond any sex at all. For me personally, I'm unable to use the word "God" without having a male image appearing before me, in the same way the word "Goddess" calls up a female image.

Just as each of us must be fully a man or woman before we

can become a "person," so too, perhaps it's appropriate for awhile to worship the Source of Our Lives with an image. But sooner or later each of us must arrive at personhood beyond our one-sex identity, and we must also worship Life as an undivided Force. Thus I also call the Source of Life: Love, Divine Love, the Life Force or Life Energy, Mercy, All-That-Is, All-the-Power-in-the-Universe, or the Beloved Source of Life.

I return briefly to sexual identity when I refer to Grace as "She." Grace is traditionally thought of as an object, not a subject, as in "God gives grace." I use the word Grace as a subject, the complement of the male "God" who's out there somewhere watching us after He created us. This seems a true parallel to nature: that the involvement of the male in the creation of life is rather distant and optional—perhaps he'll care, perhaps he won't. But the aspect of the Source of Life that stays with us to the very end is parallel to the presence of mothers in our lives. If there's an image that the world knows of never-failing concern, of love that both follows and anticipates us, surrounds us no matter whether we remember it or not—it's the mother/female archetype that belongs to those forever faithful, caring characteristics. Grace is, to me, not an object but a Presence. It upholds us not in the way food gives us strength when we eat it but in the way we feel strengthened and encouraged because someone in our lives loves us. The presence of loving people in our lives affirms us; perhaps their advice aids us, their love makes us feel stronger.

I refer to pain also as a presence, and as a loving presence with a face we don't expect and recognize. Pain is also a "she" because of its involvement in our lives, as opposed to distance. She will not be ignored; Her determination to encourage us to grow is like a mother dedicated to nurturing her children to grow into all they can be, when the child would like to be ordinary, lazy, playful, naughty. Pain is the mother who insists we grow up, and she will stick with us to see that we do.

Notes

Part I

1. Sam Keene, *Gabriel Marcel* (Richmond, VA: John Knox Press, 1968), p. 11.
2. Helen Keller, *The Story of my Life* (New York: Airmont Publishing Company, 1965), p. 46.
3. Richard Moss, "Living the Transformational Life," workshop at Oasis, Chicago, IL, March, 1989.

Part II

1. Richard Boyajian, *Where Have I Come From? Where Am I Going?* Jonathan Plummer Lecture, Illinois Yearly Meeting of the Religious Society of Friends, August 7, 1988.
2. Jane Roberts (Seth), *The Nature of Personal Reality* (New York: Bantam Books, 1988).
3. Stephen Levine, *Healing Into Life and Death* (New York: Anchor Press, Doubleday, 1987), p. 63.
4. Carlos Castaneda, *Tales of Power* (New York: Pocket Books, 1974), p. 33.
5. Elspeth Huxley, *The Flame Trees of Thika* (New York: Penguin Books, 1988), p. 264.
6. Oliver Sacks, M.D. *A Leg to Stand On* (New York: Summit Books, 1984), p. 109.
7. Michael Crichton, *Travels* (New York: Alfred A. Knopf, 1988), p. 148.
8. Castaneda, *op. cit.*, p. 19.

219

Part III

1. Stephen Levine, *op. cit.*, p. 55.

2. Oliver Sacks, *op. cit.*, p. 110.

3. Deepak Chopra, M.D., *Quantum Healing* (New York: Bantam Books, 1989), pp. 48–49.

Part IV

1. "The Greatest Love of All," sung by Whitney Huston, words by Linda Creed, music by Michael Masser, copyright 1977 by Gold Horizon Music Corporation and Golden Torch Music, Columbia Pictures Publication, 1580 N.W. 48th Avenue, Miami, FL 33014.

2. Sister Barbara Blake, written for "Wellsprings of the Creative Spirit," Mundelein College, Chicago, IL, July 8, 1987.

3. M. Conrad Hyers, quoted in Louis M. Savory and Thomas J. O'Connor, eds., *The Heart Has Its Seasons* (New York: Regina Press, 1971), p. 142.

4. "Pain and the Brain," Public Broadcasting System, November, 1988.

Part V

1. Alan Watts, *The Way of Zen* (New York: Random House Vintage Books, 1957), p. 45.

2. Stephen Levine, *op. cit.*, p. 265.

3. Stephen Levine, quoted in *The Sun* (Chapel Hill, NC: August, 1990), issue 167, p. 10.

4. Baroness Jane Ewart-Biggs, quoted in Alf McFreary, *Tried by Fire* (Basingstoke, Hampshire, U.K.: Marshall Pickering Publishers, 1981), p. 105.

5. Richard Moss, *How Shall I Live, Transforming Surgery or Any Health Crisis into Greater Aliveness* (Berkeley, CA: Celestial Arts, 1985), p. 67.

6. Oliver Sacks, *op. cit.*

7. Elizabeth Kübler-Ross, *On Death and Dying* (New York: Macmillan, 1969).

8. John Woolman, *The Journal and Major Essays of John Woolman*, ed. Phillips P. Moulton (New York: Oxford University Press, 1971), pp. 185–186.

9. Helen Keller, *op. cit.*

10. George Fox, *No More But My Love: Letters of George Fox, Quaker*, ed.

Cecil W. Sharman (London: Quaker Home Service, 1980), Epistle 206, p. 73.

11. Jacques Lusseyran, "Blindness: A New Seeing of the World," in *Parabola, the Magazine of Myth and Tradition* (New York: 1980), Vol. 5, #3, pp. 13–20.

Part VI

1. "Born Free," lyrics by Don Black, music by John Barry, Screen Gems-Columbia Music, Inc., 711 Fifth Avenue, New York, NY 10022, copyright 1966.

2. Charlotte Johnson Frisbie, *Kinaalda, A study of the Navajo Girl's Puberty Ceremony* (Middletown, CT: Wesleyan University Press, 1967), p. 189.

3. Daniel 3: 52–90

4. *Aho:* A Native American affirmation: "This is what I say; I stand behind this!"

I would like to acknowledge conversations referred to in the text with the following unidentified friends: Tom Donnelly, Natalie Kreutzer, Nancy Prise, Carol Tyx, Pauline Cheek, Tom Martish, and Sister Vivian Wilson.

Sources

The following books contributed significantly to my understanding of life and pain and so to the writing of this book. Many of these are no longer easily available, and other excellent books have been written on the topics, but what I list here is solid and worth finding. It's not the number of books we read that heals us; rather, it's the number of quality books we've eaten and digested. These I've lived with, and my life has been significantly altered for the better because of each of them.

I've listed them alphabetically under each topic (although many could be listed under several topics).

The Nature of Human Life on Earth
Bach, Richard. *Illusions, The Adventures of a Reluctant Messiah.* New York: Dell Publishing Co., Inc. 1977.
A short, delightful, modern-Jesus story with valuable insights about life and living.

Castaneda, Carlos. *Journey to Ixtlan.* New York: Pocket Books, 1976.

———*Tales of Power.* New York: Pocket Books, 1974.

———*The Second Ring of Power.* New York: Pocket Books, 1977.

———*The Eagle's Gift*. New York: Pocket Books, 1981.

———*The Fire From Within*. New York: Pocket Books, 1984.

———*The Power of Silence*. New York: Simon and Schuster, 1987.

The Castaneda books influenced me profoundly. Why? How? Ideas such as stopping the world in order to see differently, death as a guide, letting go of our old familiar identity, being open to power and guidance beyond ourselves, not making excuses, embracing life—these are a few of the important ideas presented in a captivating way.

Lao-tzu. *Tao Te Ching*, translated by Stephen Mitchell. New York: Harper & Row, Publishers, 1988. This ancient Chinese book is full of great wisdom, especially about keeping in balance, living with mystery and reverence, accepting paradoxes and opposite values.

Roberts, Jane (Seth). *Seth Speaks: the Eternal Validity of the Soul,* Bantam Books, NY, 1972.
More than anything I've ever read, the Seth books brought emotional and physical health into my life. I believe this was the first I read of the series. Seth describes us as much larger beings than we usually think, with more power than we're trained to use. He's truly at the frontier of philosophy, psychology, and science in describing what life is all about and what human consciousness is made of.

———*The Individual and the Nature of Mass Events, a Seth Book*. Englewood Cliffs, NJ: Prentice-Hall, Inc. 1981.
Seth describes how groups of people unconsciously plan events together, such as the overthrow of governments, wars, earthquakes, the emergence of new ideas.

———*The Unknown Reality*. Englewood Cliffs, NJ: Prentice-Hall, Inc. Volume One: 1977; Volume Two: 1979.

Vol 1: Consciousness is energy, no energy disappears: the road not taken was also taken. Vol 2: Atoms and cells have their own consciousness, time and space are flexible, desire and free will create all that is.

224

de Saint Exupery, Antoine. *The Little Prince*. New York: Harcourt, Brace
    & World, Inc., 1971.
The best science fiction ever written. Life on earth as freshly encountered
by an innocent child from another planet, asking the obvious questions of
what he encounters. An objective look at ourselves.

Marcel, Gabriel. *Being and Having*. Westminster: Dacre Press, 1949; also
    Fontana Library, 1965.
"Having" makes the world and other people into objects and ruins our
ability to experience even our own selves as real and living. Embracing living
is the road to holiness and enlightenment. Marcel is a philosopher: this is
not quick reading.

Buber, Martin. *I and Thou*, translated by Walter Kaufmann. New York:
    Charles Scribner's Sons, 1970.
Following Marcel, Buber presented perhaps one of the most important
concepts ever observed: the differences between I-It relationships and I-You
relationships, and the implications of choosing one or the other in our
relating with God, each other, and all creation. This is slow reading because
of the poetic language, but it's a life-changing insight.

Wilder, Laura Ingalls. *Little House on the Prairie* series. New York: Harper
    & Row, 1935.
After twice reading this series to my children, my life was never the same.
I learned much from these true stories about how to be a parent, about
facing one's challenges with joy, surviving under difficulty, caring for each
other; about happiness that comes from other than material things, about
what it means to live with quality and integrity.

Death
Kübler-Ross, Elizabeth. *On Death and Dying*. New York: Macmillan, 1969.
"The classic" and pioneering book on the natural process of dying.

Roberts, Jane. *The Afterdeath Journal of an American Philosopher, The World
    View of William James*. Englewood Cliffs, NJ: Prentice-Hall, 1978.
This channeled book is one of the most fascinating books I've ever read.
His description of what he's doing after death, what "God" is like, how he
now views what he attempted and wrote about when alive, issues of the
dead contacting the living—what he says about all these is unique.

"God"

Durka, Gloria, and Joanmarie Smith. *Modeling God, Religious Education for Tomorrow*. Paulist Press, NY, 1976.
How the images we have of God help us grow, but the images must be flexible and grow as we grow.

Driver, Tom F. *Patterns of Grace*. San Fransisco: Harper & Row, 1978.
God is affected by creation, and God changes; the universe grows forever; embracing life, the whole bag.

Stone, Merlin. *When God Was a Woman*. New York: Harcourt Brace Jovanovich, Publishers, 1976.
What's left out of history books: the evidence of the forgotten Mother religions found all over the world. Many other excellent books are now available on this topic.

Psychology

Bach, George R., and Peter Wyden. *The Intimate Enemy, How to Fight Fair in Love and Marriage*. New York: Avon, 1970.
This book helped save our marriage when we didn't know how to communicate. A wonderful book on the value and pitfalls in conflict.

Dowling, Colette. *The Cinderella Complex, Women's Hidden Fear of Independence*. New York: Summit Books, 1981.
A different kind of feminist perspective. She speaks a truth about our own part in building any patriarchical situation; the temptation to comfort and avoidance of "getting a life."

Frankl, Victor. *Man's Search for Meaning*. New York: A Kangaroo Book, Pocket Books, 1977.
A short, powerful book that helps us see a basic human need that our materialistic world has missed in our search for happiness.

Horner, Matina S. "Femininity and Successful Achievement: A Basic Inconsistency." In Judith M. Bardwick, Elizabeth Douvan, Matina Horner, and David Gutmann. *Feminine Personality and Conflict*. Belmont, CA: Brooks/Cole, 1970.
This article shook me to my depths because it spoke out loud the truth of my own suffering: holding myself back because I'm a woman.

226

Jung, Carl Gustav. *Memories, Dreams, and Relections*. New York: Random House, 1973.
Freud dealt with sick people; Jung looked also at the healthy. He opened us to a broader view of symbols and a positive view of religion, mythology, the feminine, intuitions, and many other elements of human life that Freud had judged negatively. Jung also affirms an underlying unity between our psyches. His is the broadest, healthiest view of the human psyche I'd found until the writings of Seth.

Lair, Jess, Ph.D. *Sex: If I Didn't Laugh I'd Cry*. New York: Fawcett Crest, 1979.
An old and simple book, but the healthiest I've ever read on sex and relationships.

Progoff, Ira. *The Symbolic & the Real*. New York: McGraw-Hill Book Company, 1973.
How the capacities of people can be enlarged to experience more of the fullness of life. Dr. Proghoff has also developed excellent methods of journaling for growth and change.

Roberts, Jane (Seth). *The Nature of Personal Reality*. New York: Bantam Books, 1980.
Perhaps the most personally healing and powerful of the Seth books, this is truly worth reading slowly and trying out in life: it will improve your life a hundred percent.

——*The Nature of the Psyche, Its Human Expression*. Englewood Cliffs, NJ: Prentice-Hall, Inc., 1979.
A beautiful book on relationships and the nature of sexuality.

Singer, June. *Boundaries of the Soul, the Practice of Jung's Psychology*. Garden City, New York: Doubleday, 1972.
A simple yet comprehensive description of the basic ideas of Carl Jung.

Healing

Bass, Ellen, and Laura Davis. *The Courage to Heal, A Guide for Women Survivors of Child Sexual Abuse*. New York: Harper & Row, Publishers, 1988.
For anyone trying to heal any bad memories; especially good on the value of anger, forgiveness, speaking up, moving on, the body remembers.

Field, Joanna. *A Life of One's Own*. Los Angeles: J.P.Tarcher, Inc. 1981.
The simple and honest record of the way a person healed herself into happiness by self-observation and truthfulness.

Gendlin, Eugene T. *Focusing*. New York: Bantam Books, 1982.
A simple method for getting clear about what you're feeling and learning how to say one's truth.

Levine, Stephen. *Healing Into Life and Death*. New York: Anchor Doubleday, 1987.
Healing through embracing life. Stephen and Ondrea Levine work with people who have life-threatening diseases. People's conditions are often reversed by this wonderful healing approach. Their entire view of human living is powerfully health-giving for anyone. Don't miss this.

Moss, Richard, M.D. *How Shall I Live; Transforming Surgery or Any Health Crisis into Greater Aliveness*. Celestial Arts, Berkeley, CA, 1985.
Moss integrates the spirit and body in such medical processes as surgery, taking medicine, doctor-patient relations; he sees physical crises as opportunities for transformation and growth. He gives wonderful workshops, has a good wholistic spirituality.

Sacks, Oliver, M.D. *A Leg to Stand On*. New York: Summit Books, 1984.
Dr. Sacks is a delightful and creative neurologist. This is his own story of recovery—learning to walk after a terrible accident. He's written other books about creative approaches to his patients, using natural and creative methods and observations.

Walkenstein, Eileen, M.D. *Your Inner Therapist*. Philadelphia: The Westminster Press, 1983.
A little-known, wonderful book for working with one's self, for either physical or emotional healing, using simple imagery exercises and self-dialogue.

Mindell, Arnold. *Working With the Dreaming Body*. Boston: Routledge & Kegan Paul, 1985.
How to "read" what the physical body is trying to say when it's speaking through physical symptoms.

228

Dreaming

Garfield, Patricia. *Creative Dreaming*. New York: Ballantine Books,'1974.
Simply written and comprehensive; gives an overview from many cultures
of theories and practices with dreams .

Roberts, Jane (Seth). *Dreams, Evolution, and Value Fulfillment*. New York:
 Prentice Hall, Volumes One and Two: 1986.

Vol 1: The world is constantly being created, first through dreaming.

Vol 2: Heredity and physical handicaps as positive experiments and experiences; the individual and the human species. Don't miss the Jane Roberts
books on dreaming—they go far beyond what psychologists have so far
limited themselves to.

————*Dreams and Projection of Consciousness*. Walpole, NH, Stillpoint Publishing, 1986.
Techniques for working with our subconscious; how to use dreams for
healing.

Listening

Suzuki, Shunryu. *Zen Mind, Beginner's Mind*. New York: Weatherhill, 1984.
There are many wonderful books on Zen; this is my favorite. The practice
of Zen is powerful for healing, as are many other forms of meditation.

London Yearly Meeting of the Religious Society of Friends. *Christian Faith
 and Practice in the experience of the Society of Friends*. London: Headley
 Brothers Ltd, 1988.
Like Zen, the practice of the Quakers of simple living and silent worship is
a powerful path toward getting clear inside, speaking one's truth, feeling
the presence of divine Love in one's life, and maintaining one's spiritual
bonds of unity, respect, and mutual help with all other living things.

Sources for Key Quotations

To introduce the core ideas of each meditation I've selected quotations that seemed appropriate. Here are some of the sources of these quotes:

Personal friends: Tom Forsythe, Annette Reynolds, Tom McDonald.

Carroll, Lewis. *Alice's Adventures in Wonderland*. New York: The New American Library, 1960.

Castaneda, Carlos. *Tales of Power*. New York: Pocket Books, 1974.

Erdrich, Louise. *Love Medicine*. Boston: G.K. Hall, 1986.

Forché, Carolyn. *Healing Up Morning*, in China Galand, *Longing for Darkness, Tara and the Black Madonna*. New York: Viking Penguin, 1990.

Friends Journal. Monthly publication of Friends Publishing Corporation, 1501 Cherry St., Philadelphia, PA 17331.

Greene, Alyce, and Elmer Greene. *Beyond Biofeedback*. New York: Delacourte Press/Seymour Lawrence, 1977.

Jesus of Nazareth, in Matthew 7:7 and John 8:32.

Lao-tzu. *Tao Te Ching*, translated by Stephen Mitchell. New York: Harper & Row, 1988.

Levertov, Denise. *Oblique Prayers; New Poems with 14 translations from Jean Joubert*. New York: New Directions, 1984.

Levine, Stephen. *Healing Into Life and Death*. New York: Anchor Doubleday, 1987.

Lusseyran, Jacques. "Blindness: A New Seeing of the World," in *Parabola, The Magazine of Myth and Tradition*. Vol. 5, No. 3, 1980.

Nietzsche, Friedrich. *Thus Spoke Zarathustra*, translated by R. J. Hollingdale. New York: Viking Penguin, 1969.

Paton, Alan. *Instrument of Thy Peace*. New York: The Seabury Press, 1968.

Perls, Frederick S. *In and Out the Garbage Pail*. New York: Bantam Books, Inc., 1972.

Rilke, Rainer Maria. *Poems, 1906–1926*, translated by Elizabeth Watson, in *Guests of My Life*. Burnsville, NC: Celo Press, 1979.

Roberts, Jane (William James). *The Afterdeath Journal of an American Philosopher, The World View of William James*. Englewood Cliffs, New Jersey: Prentice-Hall, 1978.

Roberts, Jane (Seth). *The Nature of Personal Reality*. New York: Bantam Books, 1988.

Roosevelt, Eleanor. Quoted in *Catholic Digest*, 1960.

Sacks, Oliver, *A Leg to Stand On*. New York: Summit Books, 1984.

Saint-Exupery, Antoine de. *The Little Prince*, translated by Katherine Woods. New York: Harcourt, Brace & World, 1971.

Watson, Elizabeth. *Guests of My Life*. Burnsville, NC: Celo Press, 1979.

Whyte, L. L., in Jamake Highwater. *The Primal Mind*. New York: New American Library, 1981.

232

If you found *PAIN: The Challenge and the Gift* meaningful and valuable, you may also wish to read:

* BREAKING FREE OF ADDICTIVE FAMILY RE-LATIONSHIPS: Healing Your Own Inner Child by Dr. Barry Weinhold

While growing up, 97% of today's adults learned from their families dysfunctional, addictive patterns from their family that often interfere with creating successful relationships. In this book, Dr. Barry Weinhold shows us how to identify and heal those destructive patterns, replacing them with healthy attitudes and behaviors.

"I heartily recommend this book. It offers practical ways to break the 'invisible loyalties' that bind us to dysfunctional families."
   —**John Bradshaw, author of Bradshaw on the Family**
   and host of the nationally televised PBS series

* BREAKING FREE OF THE CO-DEPENDENCY TRAP by Drs. Barry and Janae Weinhold

Drs. Barry and Janae Weinhold offer you effective step-by-step instructions for identifying and releasing dysfunctional and destructive relationship patterns. They challenge the widely held perception that co-dependency is permanent, progressive and incurable. They provide you with a comprehensive road map to take you from where you are—through positive change—to recovery.

"The greatest sense of hope in this book results from the precise and practical tools for recovery with which the Weinholds present us. Developmental 'stuckness' can be remedied."
   —**John Bradshaw, author of Healing The Shame That Binds You and Bradshaw On: The Family**
   and host of the nationally televised PBS series

* **CEREMONIES FOR CHANGE: Creating Personal Ritual to Heal Life's Hurts** (includes 16 full-color ritual cards)
by Lynda S. Paladin

"Through the sharing of her personal story, Lynda Paladin's symbols become real and relevant. Personal ritual for daily living proves practical and purposeful. Creative imagination, free-spirited play, and even spontaneous whimsy become genuinely meaningful. And ceremonies—elaborate or simple, are seen as sacred and deeply nourishing. This book answers a contemporary longing."
—Doug Boyd, author of Rolling Thunder
(from the foreword of the book)

Ask for these books at your favorite local bookstore or order them directly from Stillpoint by calling or writing:

Stillpoint Publishing
Meetinghouse Road, P.O. Box 640
Walpole, NH 03608
Telephone: 603-756-9281
FAX: 603-756-9282
Order Line: 800-847-4014 (except NH & outside USA)

Publisher's Note

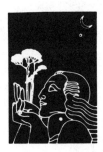

This logo represents Stillpoint's commitment to publishing books and other products that promote an enlightened value system. We seek to change human values to encourage people to live and act in accordance with a greater and more meaningful spiritual purpose and a true intent for the sanctity of all life.